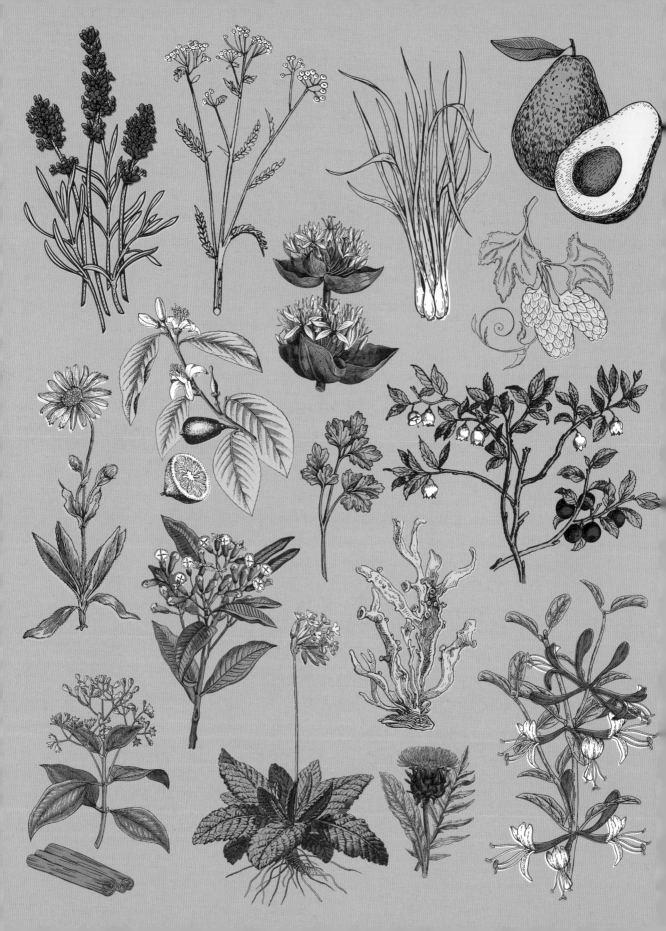

HEALING
WITH
PLANTS

*The Chelsea Physic
Garden Herbal*

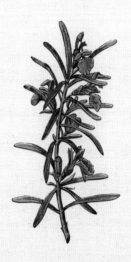

An Hachette UK Company
www.hachette.co.uk

First published in Great Britain in 2021 by Aster, an imprint of
Octopus Publishing Group Ltd
Carmelite House
50 Victoria Embankment
London EC4Y 0DZ
www.octopusbooks.co.uk

Distributed in the US by Hachette Book Group
1290 Avenue of the Americas, 4th and 5th Floors
New York, NY 10104

Distributed in Canada by Canadian Manda Group
664 Annette St., Toronto, Ontario, Canada M6S 2C8

ISBN 978 1 78325 304 3

A CIP catalogue record for this book is available from the British Library.

Printed and bound in China
10 9 8 7 6 5 4 3 2 1

Consultant Publisher: Kate Adams
Senior Managing Editor: Sybella Stephens
Copy Editor: Helen Ridge
Art Director: Juliette Norsworthy
Designer: Miranda Harvey
Picture Library Manager: Jennifer Veall
Illustrator: Ella Mclean
Production Manager: Caroline Alberti

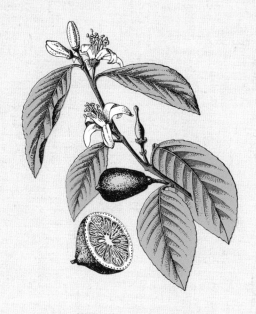

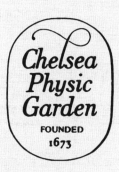

Chelsea
Physic
Garden
FOUNDED
1673

HEALING WITH PLANTS

The Chelsea Physic Garden Herbal

Written by HOLLY FARRELL

aster

CONTENTS

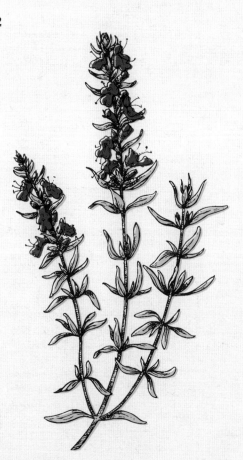

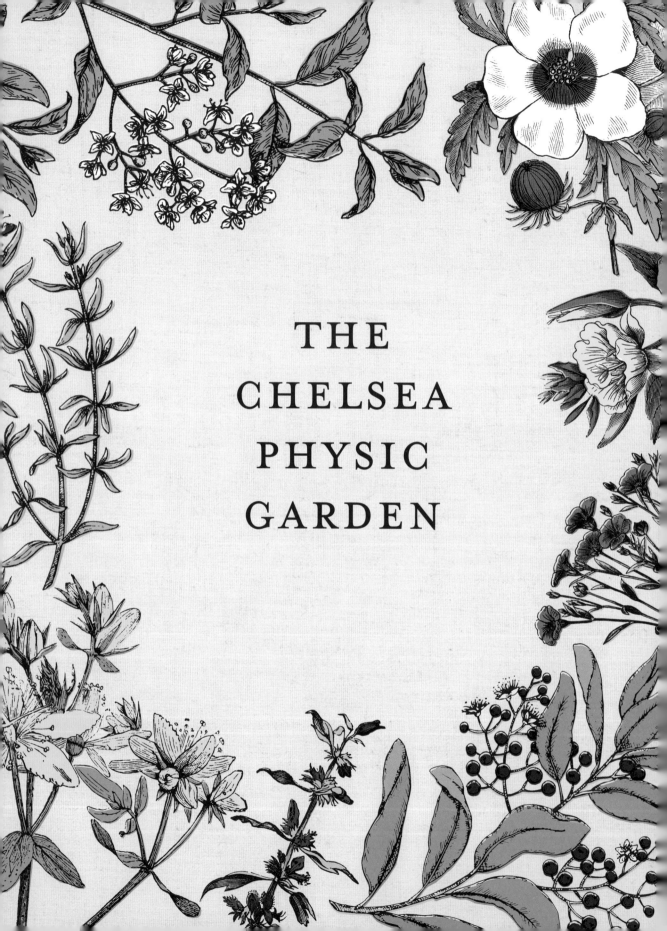

THE
CHELSEA
PHYSIC
GARDEN

THE GARDEN'S ORIGINS

Chelsea Physic Garden was founded in 1673 on land that was previously a market garden, abutting the River Thames in the then relatively rural Manor of Chelsea. The land was sheltered by walls and benefited from the warm river air, south-facing aspect and good, light soil. In short, it was an ideal spot for a garden. At that point it was simply the Apothecaries' Garden, run by the Worshipful Society of Apothecaries for growing medicinal herbs and training its apprentices how to identify and use them.

Sir Hans Sloane was one of those apprentices, and on completing his training he became the 2nd Duke of Albermarle's personal physician, travelling with him to the then English colony of Jamaica. Sloane's observations and collections incorporated many items gathered using slaves and known to the indigenous peoples including quinine, a plant-based compound that can prevent and cure malaria, and a drink using chocolate. These two discoveries, amongst others – and his marriage to an heiress of a sugar plantation - would make him a wealthy man on his return to England, when he bought the Manor of Chelsea, including the Garden. Grateful to the Society for his early training, he decreed that it could use the Garden in return for paying a sum of £5 per year in perpetuity, thus securing its future.

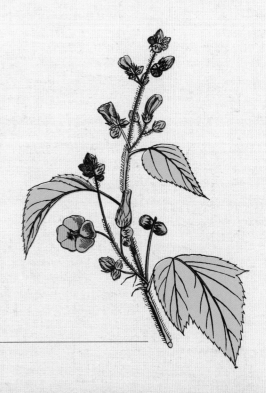

Sloane's collections of botanical and zoological specimens, libraries, manuscripts and antiquities were so vast that, when they were bequeathed to the nation on his death in 1753, the British Museum had to be built to house them, with Sloane decreeing in his will that the museum should be free to all. His herbarium (collection of dried plants), now kept at the Natural History Museum and available as an online resource, has been vital to the research of botanists for the last 300 years, including that of Carl Linnaeus (who originated the botanical Latin plant-naming system used to this day). It, like many other natural history collections of the 18th and 19th centuries, depended on the infrastructure of the transatlantic slave trade for its very existence because the regular ships crossing from the Caribbean could bring back new plants and discoveries.

WHAT IS AN APOTHECARY?

The closest modern equivalent of the 17th-century apothecary would be a pharmacist. Originally traders in herbs and spices, over time they became consultants on herbal medicine (the only medicine of the time) for the public who had no space to grow their own herbs, lacked the knowledge and/or could not afford the fees of a qualified physician. The apothecaries kept lists of the medicinal plants that they traded, and their uses and effects. By 1617 the apothecaries of Great Britain were sufficiently influential as to be allowed to incorporate by a Royal Charter, and the Worshipful Society of Apothecaries was founded. The Society continued to manage the Chelsea Physic Garden until 1899, and from 1815 to this day has regulatory powers, maintaining its position as an important medical institution.

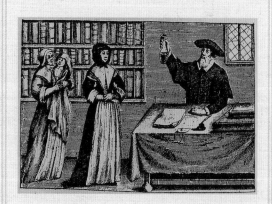

INSIDE THE CHELSEA PHYSIC GARDEN

The Garden is surrounded by brick walls on three sides, with large wrought-iron gates leading out onto Chelsea Embankment and buildings that now house offices and amenities on the northern wall. Originally the Garden would have abutted the river, to make it easier for the apothecaries to load and unload their barge for botanical expeditions and trade. The historic houses of Chelsea loom large outside the walls but entering the Garden is to step into an oasis. It is a healing garden in every sense of the word: the plants grown here illustrate the varied riches and therapeutic powers of the natural world and to spend time among them is to take a breath and enjoy a respite from the hurly-burly of the city beyond.

An incredible 5,000 different plants are grown here, including many endangered and unusual species which thrive in the Garden's microclimate. There are large specimen trees, tiny-leaved alpines on the Grade II-listed rockery, ordered beds and bountiful planters, and greenhouses ranging from the hot and humid to the damp and cool fernery.

Gardens of medicinal plants, useful plants, plants for our future and the monocotyledon and dicotyledon Order Beds, where plants are grouped by their botanical family, set out to inform, inspire and entertain. The Garden has its own horticultural trainee scheme, assists with wider research projects, and staff and volunteers lead tours, workshops and talks for the public and London's schoolchildren, all continuing Sloane's legacy to connect people with plants.

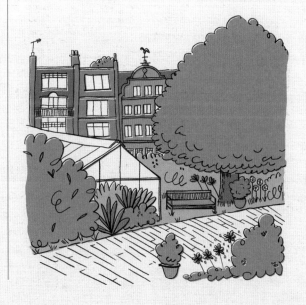

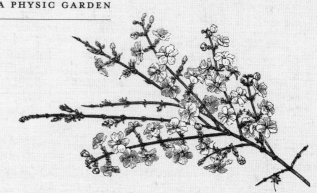

THE HEAD GARDENERS

The Garden has had many influential Curators and Head Gardeners throughout its history, many of whom have made significant contributions to the Garden and to the wider botanical and horticultural fields of knowledge.

Philip Miller, Head Gardener from 1722 to 1770, established the Garden as a centre for worldwide plant exchange and doubled the number of plant species cultivated in Britain during his tenure. His book, *The Gardeners Dictionary* (1731), was the first horticultural guide of its kind.

William Forsyth, who oversaw the garden for 13 years after Miller, was responsible for the creation of the pond rockery, the oldest surviving example of its kind in Europe.

The first half of the 19th century saw conflict between William Anderson, the Curator, and John Lindley, who held the post of Praefectus Horti, or demonstrator of plants. As medicine and botany began to diverge, Anderson wanted the Garden to become a collection of botanical curiosities, whereas Lindley was in favour of keeping it as a garden of medicinal plants. Lindley won the day, and Robert Fortune and

then Thomas Moore were appointed as Curators on his recommendation. Lindley was a significant horticultural author and professor who established the Lindley Library, the London library of horticulture now run by the Royal Horticultural Society. Lindley can also be credited with saving Kew Gardens from oblivion when the government wanted to close it in 1840.

Fortune, who presided over the Garden from 1846 to 1848, was a plant hunter extraordinaire, and was instrumental in introducing the tea plant, *Camellia sinensis*, from China to India, where it quickly became a significant national industry. He also brought back camellias and jasmine to Britain, as well as other ornamental plants that grace our gardens today, including those that bear his name such as *Trachycarpus fortunei* and *Rhododendron fortunei*. Crucial to his expeditions was the Wardian case, a portable greenhouse developed by Nathanial Ward, an associate of the Garden who used its plants to test his prototype cases. Despite his overseas adventures, Fortune still found time to establish the Order Beds, Tank Pond and glasshouses in the Garden.

Moore's tenure was not perhaps as personally significant as that of some of his predecessors, but he oversaw a time of great change in the Garden and helped lay the foundations for its future. Previously, only men had been permitted to undertake academic study of medicine and botany, but in 1877 the law changed to allow women to study plants for scientific (not medical) purposes. As medical practice continued to divest itself of natural-based healing methods, the Garden's raison d'être was being slowly erased. But as soon as women were allowed to study plants and take examinations in botany, visitor numbers jumped sixfold, with twice as many female students as male availing themselves of the Garden's plants.

The scientific study of plants gave the Garden a new purpose, and for a time in the 20th century it was a base for the Agricultural Research Council. However, it was still essentially a secret garden, a small patch of green locked away from the community. By the 1970s, both the Agricultural Research Council and the City Parochial Foundation that ran the Garden

wanted to move out. After surviving 300 years of political and financial turmoil and even the bombs of the Blitz, the Garden's future was again in peril. Once more its people came to the rescue: staff and associates, including curators Allen Paterson and Duncan Donald, raised sufficient funds to endow the Chelsea Physic Garden Company charity to keep it safe. The Chelsea Physic Garden was, finally, opened to the public in 1983.

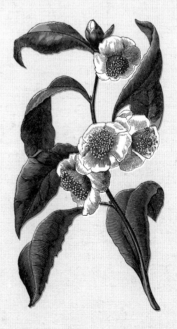

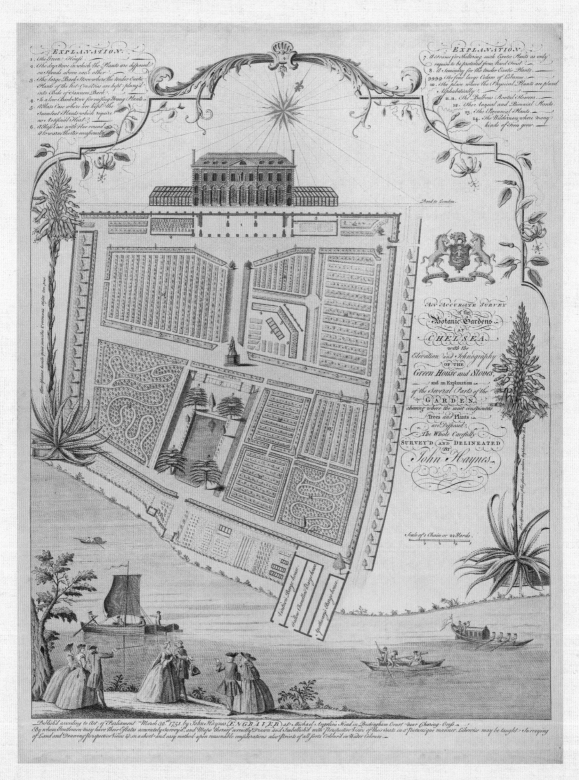

THE CHELSEA PHYSIC GARDEN TODAY

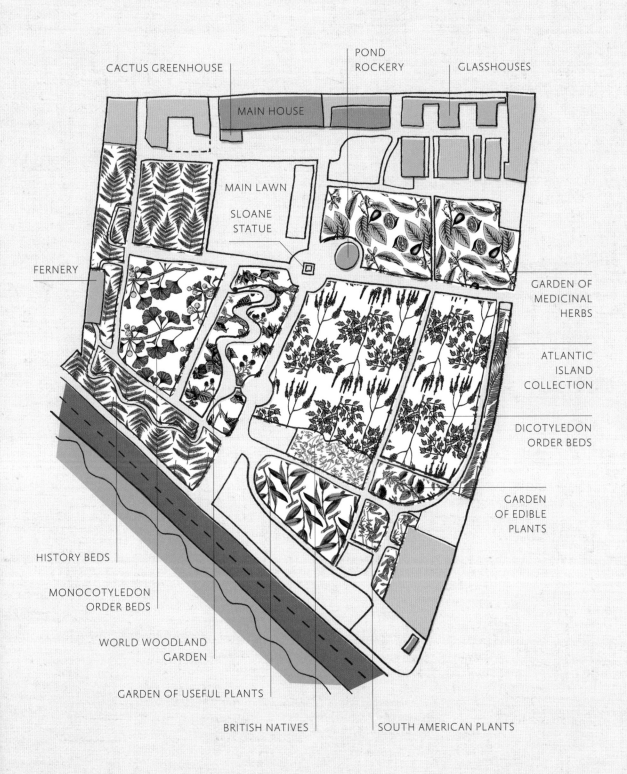

CACTUS GREENHOUSE

POND
ROCKERY

GLASSHOUSES

MAIN HOUSE

MAIN LAWN

SLOANE
STATUE

FERNERY

GARDEN OF
MEDICINAL
HERBS

ATLANTIC
ISLAND
COLLECTION

DICOTYLEDON
ORDER BEDS

GARDEN
OF EDIBLE
PLANTS

HISTORY BEDS

MONOCOTYLEDON
ORDER BEDS

WORLD WOODLAND
GARDEN

GARDEN OF USEFUL PLANTS

BRITISH NATIVES

SOUTH AMERICAN PLANTS

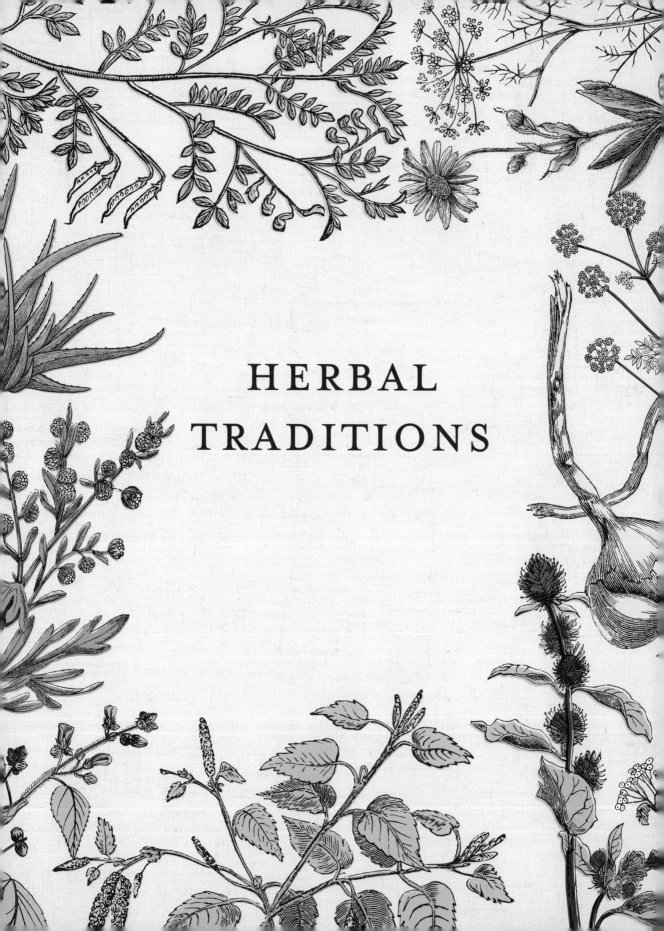

HERBAL
TRADITIONS

HERBS IN HISTORY

To follow the use of herbs through the ages is to follow the history of mankind. From the very beginning, people have used herbs as food and as medicine, imbuing them with curative, nutritive and often magical or religious qualities. Herbs have been ever present in our lives, and the earliest evidence we have is of them surrounding a Neanderthal man in a 60,000-year-old grave in Iraq. It is only in Western medicine that the connection with herbs has been lost; for 80 per cent of the world's population, herbal medicine is the only medicine. Archaeological research has also discovered that as well as using herbs in burial sites, some of the earliest humans used herbs as medicine. By the time the inhabitants of Sumer in Ancient Mesopotamia were inscribing clay tablets with herbal recipes and preparations 5,000 years ago, there were over 250 different plants that had been identified as herbs. As people migrated over land and sea, herbal traditions diversified, but like the many branches of a tree, they all share the same roots.

Western herbalism has its origins in the work of Hippocrates (*c.*460–*c.*370 BCE) and Galen (*c.*130–*c.*216 CE). Hippocrates was so influential in the founding of the medical profession that many newly qualified doctors around the world still take a version of the Hippocratic oath. According to Galen, sick people had an imbalance of four important liquids called humours (blood, black bile, yellow bile and phlegm) and the balance could be redressed through increasing or purging one or the other, often through the

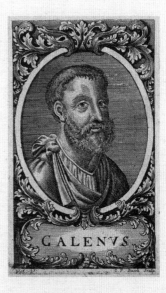

application of various herbs in isolation or combination. The idea of the body in balance, or imbalance, pervades most early herbal traditions, including Chinese medicine and Ayurveda. Other cultures use herbs in different ways. Today, tribal Amazonian medicine men diagnose patients by taking powerful hallucinogenic herbs themselves, which, combined with dancing, allows them to see the right path to health for the sufferer.

Shamanism uses herbs to drive out evil spirits from the body where they are causing illness. These many different traditions are not isolated from one another: travel by explorers, scientists or conquering armies opened up different cultures to one another and the resulting trade of ideas as well as plants led – and continues to lead – to a widening and deepening level of understanding of herbs and their properties.

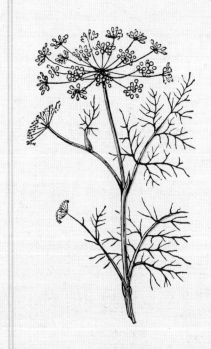

DEFINING HERBS

It is their pervasiveness in human culture that makes herbs so difficult to define. Herbs can be used for cooking (either as a food in themselves or as a flavouring), to heal, as perfume, to dye and weave fabrics, for cleaning and as natural pesticides. Botanically, a herb is a herbaceous perennial: a plant that bears seeds and has non-woody upper growth that dies back at the end of each growing season, sprouting anew the following spring. However, there are many herbaceous perennials that, while beautiful in the flower border, have no particular therapeutic application, and there are many plants that are definitely herbs (rosemary, for example) that are not herbaceous perennials. Eighteenth-century botanists gave the botanical Latin species name *officinalis* to many plants that were used by apothecaries, but again this categorization fails to include the vast majority of herbs.

In this book, a herb is taken as a plant that is therapeutically useful, either prepared as a home remedy or extracted, and used in the creation of pharmacological medicines.

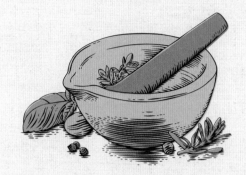

WHAT IS A HERBAL?

Herbals were *the* reference work for anyone associated with the practice of medicine for more than a millennium. From Pliny the Elder to Parkinson, essentially these books contained a list of plants with notes on each plant's identification and uses. The rhetoric of the descriptions varied wildly, from the dry and scientific, to poetic, to the downright rude and (through modern eyes) humorous, most notably in the case of Nicholas Culpeper (see page 20).

Herbals were most prominent in classical antiquity and then during the late Middle Ages, when the invention of the printing press allowed them to be reproduced far faster and more widely than by the previous painstaking copying by hand method, which also ran the risk of introducing errors. By the 16th century, physicians – who considered themselves above apothecaries, who in turn were superior to the 'herbwives' and growers of the herbs – were coming under increased criticism for their treatments, which were a great deal more expensive and generally less effective than those of country herbal healers. The study of plants and their qualities began to develop as a reaction to this, and university physic gardens began to spring up, turning botany into a respectable academic pursuit and leading to a boom in the collection, study, preservation and trade of plants.

On a domestic level, herbals were more akin to family recipe books: collections of remedies passed on from mother to daughter. Sometimes these would be kept secret, especially in the case of the village healer, who would charge for her services. Others would happily share them, such as the vicar's wife who was often responsible for the care of all those in her husband's flock, not just her own family. Also called stillroom books, herbals would be used as reminders of when and how to harvest and prepare herbs, as well as giving other useful advice for running a household, and empowered families to heal themselves in all but the most extreme cases of ill health.

NOTABLE HERBALS

Pliny the Elder was a Roman writer living in the 1st century CE. His 37-volume work *Natural History* included 16 volumes on plants, their history and usage. Pliny died at Pompeii when Mount Vesuvius erupted in 79 CE and no original version of his work survives, only monastic copies.

Dioscorides, a physician travelling with the Roman army in the 1st century CE, was so influential that herbal authors 1,500 years later were still using his *De Materia Medica* as the basis for their work, which is the reason why many herbals included

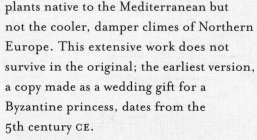

plants native to the Mediterranean but not the cooler, damper climes of Northern Europe. This extensive work does not survive in the original; the earliest version, a copy made as a wedding gift for a Byzantine princess, dates from the 5th century CE.

Medieval monasteries were among the first places to separate plants grown for healing from those for general consumption and other uses. As monasteries were also often seats of learning and had libraries, the monks would sometimes write their own works on medicine as well as copying out the classics. The polymath Hildegard of Bingen, a Benedictine abbess in 12th-century Germany who was later canonized, kept a physic garden and wrote *Physica*, a nine-volume work on the medicinal properties of plants and animals.

William Turner's *A New Herbal* (1551–68) saw him going down in history as the father of English botany, but it was closely followed by John Gerard's 1597 text. For decades Gerard's *Herball* was the predominant medicinal herbal reference

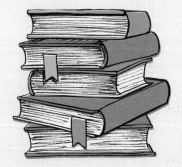

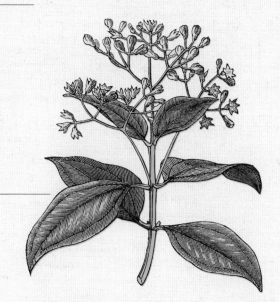

book for country households that could afford it, where families would often insert their own notes and recipes between the pages. It was unusual in that it was more of a practical guide than previous herbals, but Gerard was also a well-connected botanist able to trade information and plants with scholars and travellers at Court.

Since the ancient herbals, it had been common practice not only to accept as verbatim the prescriptions of the ancients, but also the general approach of combining as many different ingredients as possible to make a 'cure'. Thus Galene (also called Theriac and named after Galen, who conceived the potion) was a mix of innumerable herbs, animal parts and other ingredients such as viper's flesh, wine and honey, which took 40 days to prepare and was best after maturing for at least 12 years. Understandably, patients both rich and poor were beginning to tire of this quackery and the work of the Swiss-German physician Paracelsus in the early 16th century was a breath of fresh air. He scorned the herbals for their lack of original research, preferring instead

to seek out experienced country healers and wise women, and recommended using herbs simply for their specific qualities (active constituents). He also advocated the Doctrine of Signatures, the herbal system based on the idea that God marked plants to resemble the parts of the body that they should be used to heal. Thus *Pulmonaria* species, with their oval, spotted leaves resembling the lungs, should be used to treat bronchial afflictions. Their name even refers to 'pulmonary', which means relating to the lungs.

Theatrum Botanicum (1640) was John Parkinson's masterpiece. He had already written *Paradisi in Sole* (1629), literally translated as 'park-in-sun', the author's pun on his own name, the first English-language work on gardening for pleasure, aimed at the rich families among whom he worked as a royal herbalist. He was an early member of the Society of Apothecaries, and although there is no record of his having used the Garden in Chelsea, it seems likely that he would have spent time there.

Nicholas Culpeper's *The English Physician* (1653), now known as *Culpeper's Herbal*, is still in print today in its original format and with no additional notes. It was Culpeper's name that Hilda Leyel (founder of the Society of Herbalists in the UK, now the Herb Society) used for her herb shops, bringing his book to a larger audience. Culpeper was an apothecary – though he never finished his apprenticeship – who never refused a patient and made herbal medicine widely available. Allegedly his treatment success rate was so high that the medical establishment attributed his victories to witchcraft; he is reciprocally scornful of his contemporaries in his book (see below).

Sophia Grieve, known as Maud or Mrs M Grieve, was the founder of a farm and school that taught all aspects of herb growing, harvesting and selling. She was also a President of the British Guild of Herb Growers and a Fellow of the British Science Guild. Her book *A Modern Herbal* (1931) is comprehensive and detailed and now available in its entirety online.

CULPEPER QUOTES

Although much of *Culpeper's Herbal* is very similar to Parkinson's *Theatricum Botanicum*, it remains the most well known and quotable of all the medieval and renaissance herbals.

'Doctor Tradition, that grand introducer of errors, that hater of truth, lover of folly, and the mortal foe to Dr Reason, hath taught the common people to use the leaves or flowers of this plant in mouthwater, and by long continuance of time, hath so grounded it in the brains of the vulgar, that you cannot beat it out with a beetle.' (on honeysuckle)

'Common Wormwood I shall not describe, for every boy that can eat an egg knows it.'

ELIZABETH BLACKWELL'S HERBAL

The Chelsea Physic Garden is a small community, and while in its history this has been a source of conflict, it has also given rise to some heart-warming stories. In the first half of the 18th century, under the stewardship of Philip Miller, a trainee apothecary named Alexander Blackwell studied in the Garden. He later gave up medicine and started a printing business, but he fell foul of the printing Guild for operating without a licence and was thrown into debtors' prison. His wife, Elizabeth, determined to help pay the debts and secure his release, decided to create a herbal. With the support of Miller and the staff at the Garden, she illustrated the book using plants growing there, and added her husband's notes from his earlier studies. Entitled *A Curious Herbal containing five hundred cuts of the most useful Plants which are now used in the Practice of Physick; Engraved on folio Copper Plates after Drawings taken from the LIFE; To which is added a short description of ye Plants; and their common Uses in PHYSICK*, her book was produced in two volumes between 1737 and 1739.

The Garden holds a copy of *A Curious Herbal*, and prints of some of Elizabeth's illustrations can be seen around the building. The plants are presented in no particular order in the book, which gives it the feel more of a coffee-table book than a useful reference work, but there is information on each plant with a description of both its appearance and uses. The illustrations are detailed and colourful, and sometimes also include insects such as caterpillars and a rather alarming-looking mole cricket (opposite) – a species now endangered in the UK.

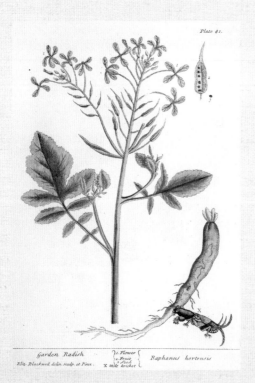

Garden Radish   *Raphanus hortensis*
Eliz. Blackwell delin. sculp. et Pinx.

HERBS IN CHINESE MEDICINE

Traditional Chinese medicine (TCM) is founded on the concept of yin and yang: yin is female, cold and dark; yang is male, hot and light. The balance between yin and yang, and between them and the five elements of wood, metal, earth, water and fire, and the flow of energy (qi) determines the state of the patient. Records of TCM exist from over 5,000 years ago. There are 300 herbal preparations listed in the *Shen Nong Ben Cao Jing* (*Divine Farmer's Classic of Materia Medica*, a 2,000-year-old Chinese text on agriculture and plants); today the TCM pharmacopoeia lists more than 2,000 remedies. Many herbs are taken as tonics to maintain the body in balance rather than to treat complaints when they occur. Ginseng is a key tonic herb in TCM.

HERBS AND MAGIC

Plants – and herbs in particular – are closely intertwined with folklore and ritual and thus, inevitably, magic. Wherever there is a lack of understanding as to how something works, there is the tendency to attribute it to magic, which is why so many medieval women who used herbs to treat the sick were accused of witchcraft. To this day, many who identify as herb witches or white witches attribute magical powers to plants, which they use to brew potions to fulfil the heart's desire. This can have an unfortunate detrimental effect on the reputation of healing plants, with those of a more scientific disposition lumping all herbal preparations – the mystical and the more grounded – into one and dismissing them out of hand.

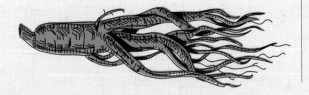

AYURVEDA AND HERBAL MEDICINE

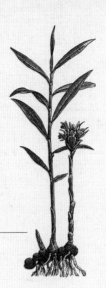

Ayurveda, meaning 'science of life', has been the herbal tradition of healing on the Indian subcontinent for at least the last 4,000 years. It describes the patient as a microcosm of various forces and elements similar to those in TCM (see opposite). In Ayurveda, prana (breath, or life), agni (spirit, or fire) and soma (love, or harmony) interact with the elements of earth, fire, water, air and ether by flowing through energy centres (chakras) in the body. A herbal prescription would depend on the imbalance of these and the profile of the humours (vata – wind; pitta – fire/bile; kapha – phlegm) in the patient.

For example, ginger stimulates agni in the body and is therefore useful against kapha illnesses, such as coughs and congestion.

Ayurveda deals with the physical body and includes prescriptions for herbal medicine, diet, exercise, surgery and psychology. The overall emphasis is to keep the body as healthy and balanced as possible to enable the body to fight disease by itself and promote healing; other aspects of the Vedic approach include yoga, meditation and astrology. Where illnesses arise, treatments aim to rebalance the body, addressing the problem's cause rather than suppressing its symptoms.

QUACKS

As medicine moves away from plant-based remedies, the term 'quack' has been applied to herbalists. There have always been those who prey on the sick, taking advantage of their worries and weakness, and charismatic yet charlatan healers who dispensed useless or downright dangerous preparations were historically commonplace. A 'quack' was a person who sold remedies knowing full well that they would not work, although the term has also been used by the medical profession to describe anyone, particularly unqualified persons, promoting treatments of which they disapprove. The word 'quack' derives from the early Dutch *quacksalver*, meaning someone who quacks on (boasts) about their salves (healing lotions and other preparations).

OTHER USES OF HERBS FOR HEALING

Homeopathy is not the same as herbal medicine. It uses minute doses of herbs that, in larger doses, would replicate the ailment they are being used to treat: the idea is that 'like cures like'. It is a holistic approach that takes into account lifestyle factors and patient history.

Aromatherapy uses the essential oils of herbs to promote physical and mental well-being. A treatment usually includes a consultation, the blending of relevant essential oils (for example, lavender for relaxation, antiseptic tea tree to fight infection, or peppermint to help the digestion) and the massaging of those diluted oils into the skin for absorption by the body.

The Bach Flower Remedies are preparations made according to the directions set down by Dr Edward Bach in the 1930s, to harness the individual spirits or energies of the 38 plants that Bach identified as being beneficial to emotional balance. Each remedy corresponds to a particular emotion, and can be taken individually or combined to support the health of the patient.

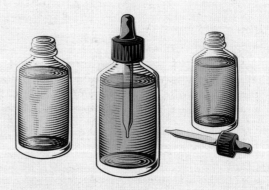

MODERN HERBALISM AND WESTERN MEDICINE

Once particular compounds were extracted from plants – for example, opium from poppies – in the 19th century, Western herbal medicine was well on the road to transforming into conventional medicine. However, in conventional medicine, it is thought that around 40 per cent of drugs are still plant-based, and some extracts from living plants are still more effective than synthesized versions. Studies have shown that extracts from snowdrops and daffodils (both toxic in their entirety) have been effective against the symptoms of Alzheimer's disease, and anticancer compounds have been found in the Madagascar periwinkle and yew trees. Modern pharmacology is screening and testing plants for their individual components, which can fluctuate depending on factors such as location and season. As habitats are destroyed and extinction before discovery is a real possibility, 'sacred groves' are being established to protect sites of special scientific interest.

In order to practise today, herbalists should have a qualification in herbal medicine, and they are also subject to the laws in the country in which they practise (which may prohibit them from actually dispensing). Where a pharmacologist would isolate a particular compound from a plant, a herbalist would prescribe the whole plant because its many different constituents work together – synergistically – to have a healing effect, often with a lower risk of side-effects or toxicity than conventional drugs. For example, where the pharmacologist might isolate salicylic acid from meadowsweet to make aspirin for pain relief, the herbalist would infuse meadowsweet flowers to make a pain-relieving drink.

Healing herbs have a significant role in the growing interest in the connection between what we eat and our overall health. This has led to some clinical trials, but for those remedies not yet empirically proven effective, there is still centuries' worth of anecdotal evidence of their efficacy. Using healing herbs empowers us to take responsibility for our own health. All the herbal traditions emphasize the need for a balanced lifestyle and a holistic approach to health and well-being, and they use herbs in the support of that everyday aim.

HEALING HERBS

The intention and culmination of all the work of the botanists, plant hunters, physicians and gardeners of the physic gardens was that the herbs they discovered and cultivated were used therapeutically. Herbal preparations were medicine for thousands of years, yet with the advent of modern medicine, the knowledge and confidence to use herbs in everyday life has been mostly lost. Recipes and tips that our great-grandparents knew have not been passed down to generations unable or unwilling to use herbs to complement a healthy lifestyle.

Herbalists use all manner of herbs in isolation or combination to treat their patients holistically. The tips and recipes given in this herbal are just an introduction to the subject, and for more information and detail it is best to consult a qualified herbalist or undertake a course in herbalism. However, the 'folk' method of herbalism – that is, the simple preparations that were and are practised by ordinary folk rather than herbal physicians and that involve no complicated measurements – is as basic as brewing a tisane of fresh mint, and brings healing herbs to everyday life.

A NOTE ON PLANT NAMES

For those new to plants and gardening, the botanical Latin names (such as those on the plant labels at Chelsea Physic Garden) can be off-putting but there is a very good reason for them. They are used because they are both unique and universal, unlike the common names of plants, such as elder, hawthorn and fennel, which can vary not only between countries but also within a country. A plant can have many different common names, and different plants can have the same common name, whereas botanical Latin names are the only version of that name given to the plant. Thus gardeners all over the world can talk to each other and be sure they are referring to the same plant.

All botanical Latin names follow the same format: the genus (plural: genera) name followed by the species. These can then be followed by variety or subspecies names at the end. For example, thyme's botanical Latin name is *Thymus vulgaris* (the Latin is always italicized): there are many different types of thyme, all grouped in the genus *Thymus*, but only this particular plant is given the species name *vulgaris*. Genera of plants that bear similar characteristics are grouped into families, and while this is not always used on labels, it can be a useful identification tool. Many herbs, such as lavender, rosemary and thyme, are in the family Lamiaceae, and all genera in this family share characteristic square stems. The species and common names are also often informative as to the plant's appearance, origins or uses.

As advances are made in DNA mapping and plant cataloguing, this sometimes means plant names will change. For example, rosemary, which was called *Rosmarinus officinalis*, was found to have more in common with the *Salvia* genus and so it has recently been renamed *Salvia rosmarinus*. Common names are generally used for everyday conversation, but it is good to have the botanical Latin to hand for certainty in identification.

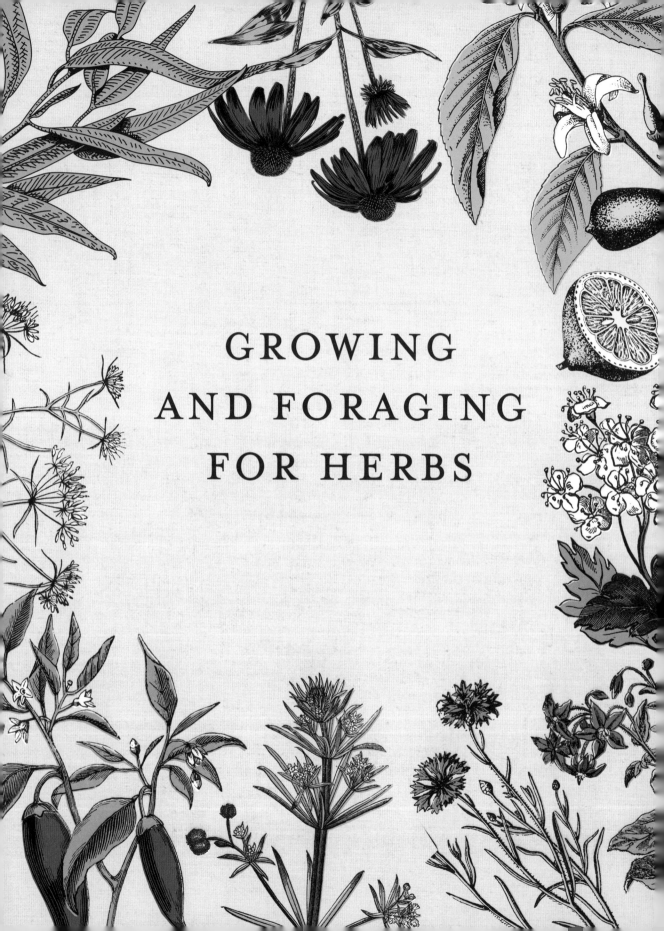

GROWING
AND FORAGING
FOR HERBS

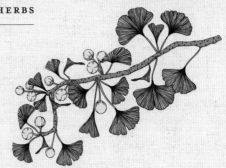

CREATING A HEALING GARDEN

Gardening is a powerful tool for healing the body and promoting good health. The simple act of going outside, breathing fresh air and touching the plants and soil can create a wealth of health benefits. These include increased serotonin levels; higher levels of invigorating oxygen entering the lungs (compared with stale indoor air); a strengthened immune system; and an increased diversity of gut flora. Then there are the cardiovascular, muscle-strength and flexibility benefits from gardening as a gentle form of exercise. Nurturing plants also brings with it an increased sense of mental well-being and can help to alleviate symptoms of depression and anxiety. The nectar from flowers and habitats provided by growing even just a few plants can also be enormously beneficial to wildlife, which in turn provides diversion and pleasure for the gardener.

Creating a healing garden thus has a two-fold beneficial effect: growing plants is good for us, and growing plants that are intrinsically healing means we can also reap the benefits of the harvest in our diet.

'Here's fine rosemary, sage and thyme. Come, buy my ground ivy.
Here's featherfew, gilliflowers and rue. Come, buy my knotted marjoram, ho!
Come, buy my mint, my fine green mint. Here's fine lavender for your cloaths,
Here's parsley and winter savory, And heartsease which all do choose.
Here's balm and hyssop and cinquefoil, All fine herbs it is well known.
Let none despise the merry, merry cries of famous London Town.'

The Cries of London, a 17th-century English ballad collected in the *Roxburghe Ballads* (1847)

DESIGNING A HEALING GARDEN

Creating a garden should not be a daunting task. Gardens are immensely personal places, a piece of ground into which the gardener pours their soul to create their own sanctuary, somewhere they can simply be. It could be outside the back door or tucked away like a secret garden; it could contain a calming water feature or be just somewhere to sit, or a forest garden or a wildflower meadow. It matters not. It is a healing place for you.

A PLAN FOR A HEALING GARDEN

The herb patch design (opposite) is only 2m (6½ft) wide by 3m (10ft) long, yet shows how many healing herbs can be grown in a small space. The plants are all perennials, with the exception of the angelica, and have been chosen for their useful healing properties for both mind and body.

View the front of this design from the right-hand side: the lower-growing chamomile should be at the front edge and the taller fennel and angelica at the back. A central path – or stepping stones – allows for regular access to harvest the herbs without unduly compacting the soil.

For the digestion:
· angelica · chamomile · fennel
· meadowsweet · peppermint

For women's health:
· angelica · lady's mantle · lemon balm
· rose

For immune-boosting and antibacterial properties:
· echinacea · lemon balm · lavender
· rosemary

To soothe and calm the nerves:
· lavender · lemon balm · rose

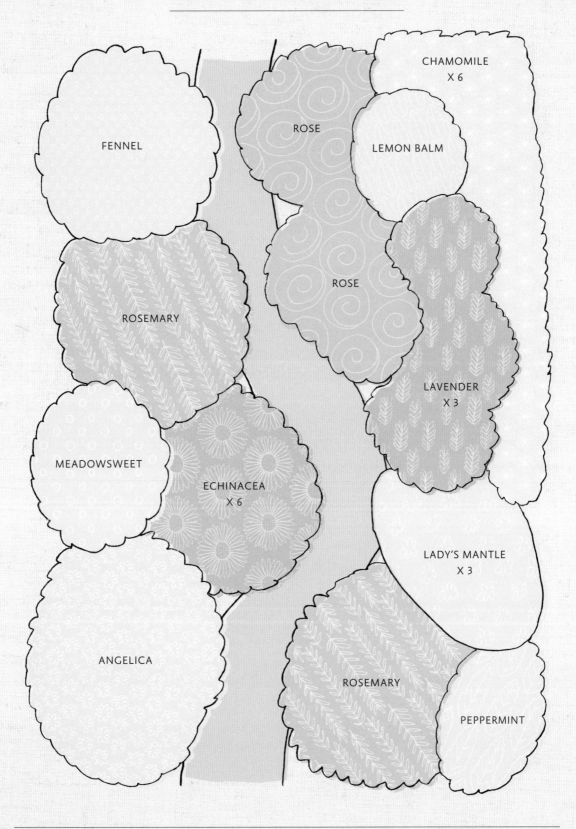

FENNEL

CHAMOMILE
X 6

ROSE

LEMON BALM

ROSE

ROSEMARY

LAVENDER
X 3

MEADOWSWEET

ECHINACEA
X 6

LADY'S MANTLE
X 3

ANGELICA

ROSEMARY

PEPPERMINT

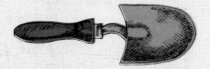

GROWING HERBS

Growing one's own herbs is the only way to guarantee their quality and provenance. Allotments, community gardens or garden-shares are all great alternatives when growing space at home is tight or non-existent. For herbs to flourish, they should be given the growing conditions that are as near as possible to those of their native habitat. Thus a rosemary plant, suited to rocky Mediterranean scree, will not do well in a waterlogged, shady border, and turmeric, a tropical rainforest-dweller, will die if left outside in the cold winter and is more suited to being grown as an indoor pot plant.

IN THE GROUND

It is easy to judge the soil type with a quick test. Scoop a small handful of damp soil. If it is easily shaped into a ball, the soil tends towards the clay end of the scale: if it can then be rolled into a sausage, the higher the proportion of clay. Damp soil that feels (and looks) gritty and is not easily moulded tends towards the sandy end of the scale. Assess, too, how many stones or even rubble there is in the soil, and how dark and rich it looks, which indicates how much compost or organic matter, for example, well-rotted manure or leaf mould, has been added. The more clay and organic matter in the soil, the more easily it will hold onto moisture and nutrients that can then be taken up by the plants; the reverse is true for sandy, stony and poor soils. Ensuring that the soil drains adequately (meaning that it is not boggy in wet weather) and is given an annual application of compost/organic matter will be enough to support the majority of herbs that grow outside in a temperate climate, but refer to the individual plants' requirements.

Before planting, if the ground is compacted – for example, if it was previously lawn – fork over the soil and turn in plenty of compost/organic matter. Remove any large stones and weeds at the same time. Consolidate it again by shuffling over it (like a penguin!), to remove the larger, undesirable air pockets, and rake level.

OUTSIDE IN POTS

Many herbs are well suited to growing in pots, but always give a plant as big a pot as possible. This will not only save on watering time (more potting compost holds more water and for longer) but also allows space for a healthy root system. Ensure the pot has adequate drainage holes and leave a gap of about 2cm (1in) at the top of the pot so the compost does not flow over the sides during watering.

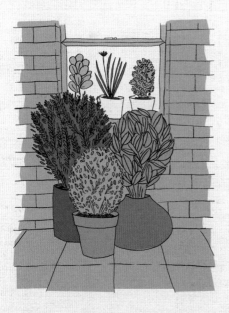

HERBS AS HOUSE PLANTS

Tropical and frost-tender herbs can sometimes be grown as house plants, depending on the available space and light levels. They may not flower or fruit as they would in their native habitat, but they can still make good (edible) foliage plants. For example, cardamom has lovely fragranced leaves, and the leaves of turmeric can be used for wrapping vegetables or fish for cooking, to impart a delicious flavour. Coffee and chocolate make interesting and attractive house plants, while pelargoniums and hibiscus are better grown indoors than out in temperate climates.

Always ensure the pot is not sitting in a pool of water. Put the plants in the best possible position for their requirements, ensuring they are not in a draught or the drying airflow from radiators. House plants benefit from being turned regularly to ensure even growth, and in the summer, if possible, move the plants outside once all risk of frost has passed. Water and feed regularly, and repot annually to keep them healthy.

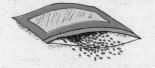

GROWING HERBS FROM SEED

Growing plants from seed can be an inexpensive and highly satisfying way to create a herb garden, but there are a number of caveats. First, those herbs that grow as shrubs or trees will take many years to reach a decent size when harvesting would be possible. Second, some varieties of herbs do not come true from seed, and so are simply not available to buy. However, for growing annual and perennial herbs, seeds are available either from garden centres or specialist herb growers. The precise method for each particular plant will vary slightly, so refer to the seed packet for more sowing information. In general, seeds are sown in spring, with each seed buried at a depth twice its size.

BUYING HERB PLANTS

For the more impatient gardener, or for shrubs and trees, herbs can also be bought as young or mature plants. The most common can be found in garden centres and even supermarkets, but for quality and more unusual species, it is usually necessary to go to a specialist herb nursery either in person or online. Choose stocky, healthy-looking plants with no sign of pests or disease damage, and a well-developed root system in the pot (tip it out to check). When making online purchases, ensure the vendor has a no-quibbles return policy.

'Here'e flowers for you,
Hot lavender, mints, savory, marjoram,
The marigold that goes to bed wi' the sun,
And with him rises weeping.'

William Shakespeare, *The Winter's Tale* (1609–11)

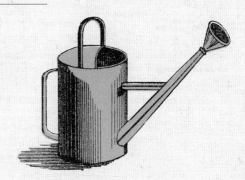

WATERING

Easily the most basic of garden tasks and yet the one that so many new gardeners find nerve-wracking, watering is necessary for most plants at some point, and essential for anything grown in a pot. It's a chance to check in with the plants and just be among them, and watering confidence will grow with experience. Some herbs need specialist watering treatment, but in general the information below is true of all plants.

SEEDS

Water the potting compost before sowing the seeds, or they can get washed away. Thereafter, keep the compost damp using a rose on the end of a watering can or a spray bottle.

POTTED PLANTS

From young seedlings to small trees, any plant grown in a pot will need regular watering, sometimes twice daily in hot conditions. Check the moisture level of the potting compost by poking a finger into it. It should feel damp but not sodden.

If it is sodden, it needs no water; if it is dry, water it now. Water in short bursts so that the water has a chance to sink in before the next application. Stop when it begins to run from the base of the pot.

PLANTS GROWING IN THE GROUND

New plantings will need a good soak after planting and regularly (daily if it's hot, dry and/or windy) thereafter until they have put out roots into the surrounding soil. Established plants will also need help with extra watering in prolonged dry periods – check the soil and water as above.

Water in the mornings or evenings where possible, and always soak everything as much as possible rather than giving an ineffectual quick splash on the surface. Direct the water to around the base of the plants, where the roots are, not onto the foliage.

FERTILIZING

Most soils will have sufficient nutrients for the plants growing in them, provided they are annually dressed with a layer of compost or other organic matter. Plants grown in pots will quickly exhaust the nutrients in their potting compost and therefore need extra nutrients. This can be in the form of controlled-release (often called slow-release) pellets or a liquid fertilizer, which will give a more immediate boost. Organic options include liquid seaweed or a homemade comfrey leaf infusion. For the latter, half-fill a bucket with comfrey leaves (see page 221); weigh them down with a brick then fill the bucket with water. Cover with a board and leave for 3–4 weeks, then strain and dilute with more water at a ratio of 1 part comfrey liquid to 4 parts water before applying to the plants. This can be repeated weekly through the growing season; the soaked leaves can be composted.

PRUNING & CUTTING BACK

Pruning is removing branches or stems of woody plants to reduce their size, keep them healthy and/or to promote flowering or fruiting. For example, lavender plants are pruned every year after flowering to remove the old flower stalks and some of the new growth to prevent the plant from becoming straggly and unsightly. Pruning should be carried out throughout the year, depending on the plant and its requirements.

Cutting back is the removal of dead stems and stalks from herbaceous perennials (plants whose foliage dies back every autumn but whose roots persist and shoot anew in spring). Pruning can be carried out in autumn, once the plant's top growth has died back. However, these stems are valuable winter shelter for insects, and the seedheads a feast for birds (not to mention good for winter flower arrangements and attractive in the frost), so where possible leave this until late winter, cutting the stems back to the base before the new shoots appear.

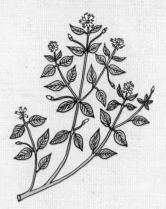

WEEDING

A weed is, as the adage goes, a plant in the wrong place. This is especially true in the herb garden, where many plants that other gardeners consider weeds are actually herbs – for example, nettles, chickweed, plantain and dandelions – which can be harvested rather than composted. However, some plants are particularly adept at spreading themselves around and can quickly colonize a garden, out-competing other plants, so some control is necessary. As with all gardening, weeding is a chance to be out among the plants – and where better to weed than a herb garden, with the scents of the foliage rising and mingling as one works among them. A little regular attention is more efficacious than sporadic weeding marathons.

Annual weeds grow quickly, setting seed in the same season. Control them by ensuring they do not set seed, which could be by harvesting all the flowers for drying or for immediate use and/or by pulling them up – they usually have a shallow root system.

Perennial weeds will return year on year from the same plant and in order to remove them, they need to have all their roots dug up from the soil, which should then be burned or dried out until they are completely dead before composting. Some plants have especially pernicious root systems that will resprout from tiny pieces of root left in the soil, such as bindweed, horsetail and ground elder, and so need regular attention to eventually weaken the plant enough to remove it from that section of soil.

'What is a weed? A plant whose virtues have not yet been discovered.'

Ralph Waldo Emerson, *Fortune of the Republic* (1878)

FORAGING FOR HERBS

Gathering herbs from the wild to nourish and heal our bodies also nourishes our souls by connecting us with nature, wildlife, folklore and history. Many herbs can be found growing in hedgerows, woodlands, parks and alongside paths, rivers and canals. Foraged herbs are particularly useful when it comes to the larger trees and shrubs such as hawthorn and elder – plants that may be too large to grow in the garden but are common enough in the wild. Start by learning to identify the plants and the richness of the natural world will soon become apparent.

When foraging for herbs from the wayside or other land, be sure to collect within common-sense safety guidelines, that is, be mindful of the surroundings and potential risks. It's best not to pick herbs growing within the first few feet of a roadside or those that are potentially mud- or urine-splattered. If possible, avoid collecting near heavy traffic, as polluting particulates and dust can coat leaves, flowers and stems. The same is true of collecting near farmland where plants could be contaminated with the drift from chemical fertilizers or pesticide sprays.

IDENTIFYING PLANTS

The first step to gathering herbs from the wild is to learn to identify them. There are many guidebooks on wildflower, tree and shrub identification, so use one or more of these, taking them out regularly with you on walks. Observe the leaves, bud arrangement, flowers, stem shape and colour, as well as the growth habit of the plant to make a positive identification. There are often many species and varieties of the same plant, and different plants known by the same common name, so be sure that you have the right one by referring to the botanical Latin name (see page 27). If there is any level of doubt, do not pick the plant. Many herbs are easily confused with other completely different plants, some of which are poisonous. A foraging course can also be a useful starting point, but confidence will come with experience and practice.

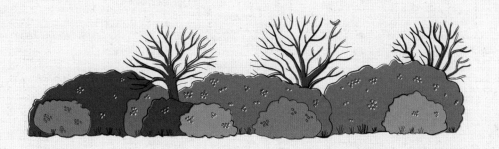

TAKE ONLY WHAT YOU NEED

When gathering herbs from the wild, it is important to harvest sustainably, leaving a good portion of the plant for wildlife and other foragers. Pick a little from several plants, rather than a lot from a single plant, and never more than half of what is there; if there is only one plant, take only a small fraction of it. Decimating a plant can weaken it, resulting in a poorer harvest the following year or even the plant's death.

FORAGING AND THE LAW

Check the local foraging bylaws before going to parks and other municipal land. On common land in the UK it is acceptable to forage for flowers, fruit, foliage and fungi for personal consumption only – it is not permitted to dig up any plants or harvest their roots. Plants on private land and farmland, for example land owned by the National Trust or the Forestry Commission, are the property of the landowner, so always ask for permission or check the relevant website.

BUYING DRIED HERBS

When growing or foraging for herbs is impossible, you can buy them already dried from herbal shops and online. Reputable vendors will have an open and transparent sourcing policy and sell dried herbs that should smell vibrant (not musty) with a good colour. Some herbs are over-exploited in the wild, so be sure that the vendor operates only with sustainable farmers and foragers; they should be able to tell you the botanical Latin name of the herb and when it was harvested and dried. Many herbal shops will also sell waxes, oils and bottles with which to make herbal preparations.

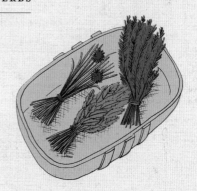

HARVESTING HERBS

For maximum potency, herbs should be harvested at their peak:

• Check the plant is not infested with pests or infected with disease – look particularly on the undersides of leaves for aphids and mould and use only fresh-looking, green foliage in good condition.

• Flowers should be newly opened, fragrant and full, not browned at the edges.

• Follow the foraging guidelines on pages 38–9 if applicable.

• Get to know how different growing and weather conditions affect the texture, fragrance and taste of the herbs because this can vary between even two plants in the same garden. Take notes to refer back to the following year and/or to amend growing practices.

'Next resolution: use your eyes, both in other people's gardens and in your own…The more you observe and take in, one way or another, the more intensely you are living and the younger you will keep in mind, if not in body.'

Christopher Lloyd, *Cuttings: A Year in the Garden with Christopher Lloyd* (2008)

DRYING HERBS

It is possible for many herbs to be preserved by drying so that they can be used throughout the year. To dry small or delicate parts of the plant, lay them out on a piece of muslin or a clean, dry cloth or tea towel and leave to dry in a warm and dry place with good air circulation, such as on a sunny windowsill or in an airing cupboard. Longer stems can be tied into small bunches and hung upside down in a similarly warm, dry place. For hard, tough stems, roots and berries, dry them on a tray lined with baking paper in an oven on its lowest setting with the door propped open. This can take several hours, so larger pieces are best sliced before drying. Once the herbs are completely dry, store in an airtight container in a cool dark place. Label the container with the plant name and the dates of harvesting and storing.

Leaves and flowers are best used within a year; stems, roots and berries within two years. Check every time the container is opened that the herbs still smell fresh and vibrant (not musty), and there should be no signs of damp or mould. Discard batches that are contaminated in this way. Note how quickly the herbs run out and grow/forage more or less next year as appropriate, or supplement with bought herbs (see page 39).

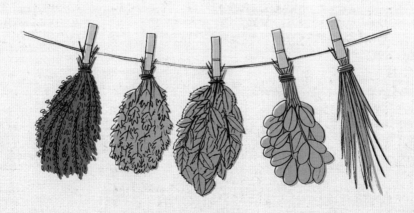

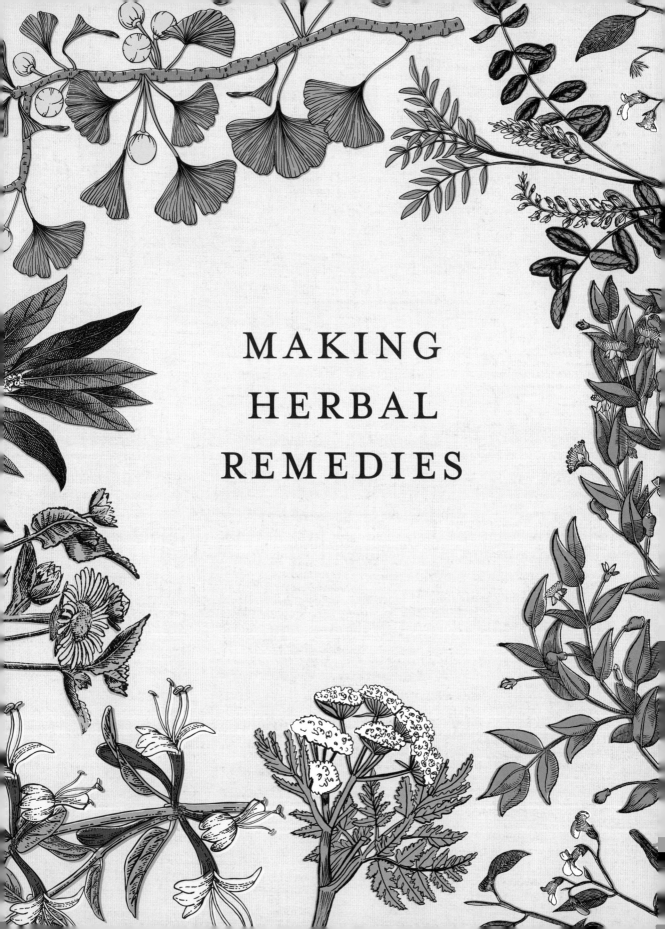

MAKING HERBAL REMEDIES

USING HERBS SAFELY

Using herbs as part of a holistic approach to balanced health and to treat minor ailments is something that is not only achievable but also immensely empowering and satisfying, not to mention calming in the creative act of just making the remedy.

The suggestions for herb uses given in this book are based on age-old remedies for self-help in the case of minor injury and illness, and to support overall health. The information is intended to educate and inspire, and is not a means of self-diagnosis or treatment. Any home-made preparations should be taken with caution (for example, patch-test any external preparations), never to excess, and only when the herbs have been identified with complete certainty (see also page 27). Consult a qualified herbalist and/or a doctor if in doubt and always in the case of chronic or severe illness or when taking long-term medication.

Herb preparations are not advisable for pregnant or breastfeeding women, or children under the age of two. For children under the age of 14, seek professional advice and adjust the dosage of each preparation accordingly.

Essential oils should never be consumed.

GENERAL NOTES ON MAKING HERBAL REMEDIES

Always wash and sterilize jars and bottles before using them to store preparations. Either wash the jars, dry and then place them in an oven warmed to 100°C (212°F) for at least 15 minutes, or put them through a 90°C (194°F) cycle in the dishwasher. Ensure they are completely dry before using.

To strain herbs from infused water, oil or syrups, use a fine sieve. For finely chopped or crumbled dried herbs, you may need to line the sieve with muslin, which is available from home-preserving suppliers and sometimes sold as 'jelly bags'.

Store preparations and dried herbs in a cool, dry and dark place – use brown, blue or green glass bottles to help preserve them.

WATER-BASED INFUSIONS

Often called the 'universal solvent', water can dissolve and extract more substances than any other liquid and is readily available, making it a natural choice for infusing many herbs. There are several types of simple water-based infusions: hot and cold infusions, decoctions and herbal baths.

To prepare a hot-water infusion:
Hot-water infusions are also known as tisanes or fresh herbal teas. The word 'tea' is widely but inaccurately applied here; strictly speaking, a tea contains the leaves of *Camellia sinensis* (the tea plant, see page 99) either in black or green form. The terms 'hot-water infusion' and 'tisane' are used interchangeably in this book.

Put 1 teaspoon of dried herbs per person (or 2–3 teaspoons of fresh herbs) into a teapot or French press. Tearing the leaves of fresh herbs will help to release their constituents. Pour over around 250ml (1 cup) of just-boiled (not boiling) water and put on the lid. Leave to infuse for 5 minutes before straining and pouring.

It is also possible to make the infusion straight into a cup, using a tea strainer or by fishing out the herbs with a fork at the end, but be sure to cover the cup with a saucer while it infuses, otherwise the beneficial herbal oils will escape with the steam.

For a stronger flavour, make a long hot-water infusion. Prepare as above but leave the herbs to infuse for 4–12 hours – after 4 hours move the infusion to the fridge – then strain.

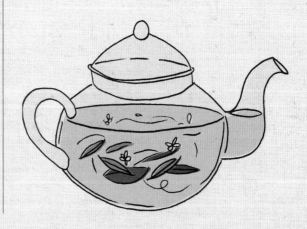

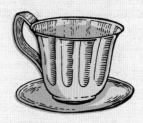

To prepare a cold-water infusion:
Some herbs, especially leafy greens and demulcent (mucilaginous) herbs, respond better to infusion in cold water, typically as a long infusion, and make a refreshing summer drink.

Put 2–3 teaspoons of dried herbs or a handful of fresh herbs into a glass bottle, large jar, jug or pitcher. Tearing and/or bashing fresh herbs using a pestle and mortar helps to release the constituents of the herbs. Cover with 500–600ml (2–2½ cups) of cold water and leave in the fridge for 4 hours or overnight to infuse. Sealed jars can be left on a sunny windowsill for the infusion time where the sunlight will help to steep the herbs. Strain into a clean glass to serve, with a few new sprigs of the herb and slices of lemon, orange and/or cucumber.

To prepare a decoction: Tough plant material, such as bark, roots and berries, needs more heat to help break it down. Put 1–2 teaspoons of plant material into a small, lidded saucepan and pour over 250ml (1 cup) of cold water. Cover with the lid and bring to a boil over a medium heat, then reduce to a simmer. Simmer for 10–20 minutes, depending on the toughness of the material, then strain.

To prepare a herbal bath: One of the most relaxing ways to use herbs, fragrant flowers and leaves is in a warm, soothing bath, where they impart their healing properties.

Strew the running bath with a handful or two of the herbs, or tie them up in a cloth bag (muslin or cotton) and suspend it under the running tap. (If strewing, it pays to have a strainer over the plughole to collect the herbs and avoid blocking pipes when emptying the bath.) Larger volumes of cold- and hot-water infusions and decoctions can also be poured into a bathtub for a similar effect. Add Epsom salts, too, if desired.

TINCTURES

Tinctures are infusions of herbs in alcohol, which preserves the herbs. A tincture can keep for up to two years, compared with just 24 hours for an infusion. The concentration of herbs is stronger, so the dosage is much smaller (1 teaspoon at a time, up to three times a day).

To prepare a tincture: Fill a glass jar with the chosen herbs, tearing up the leaves and stems of fresh plants. Pour over the alcohol – vodka with a minimum 40 per cent ABV (80 per cent proof) is ideal, but brandy or rum of the same strength can also be used – ensuring all the herbs are submerged. Screw the lid on tightly, and label with the date and contents. Leave to steep for 2–4 weeks in a cool, dark place, giving the jar a shake every other day or so. Strain the herbs and store the tincture in a clean bottle, making sure to label it with the date and contents.

For tinctures made with tougher plant material, such as roots, bark and so on, make a decoction (see page 45) of the herbs first, simmering until the liquid is reduced by half. Measure the liquid (including the plant material) and add an equal volume of alcohol, mix and pour into a jar to steep. Strain and store as above.

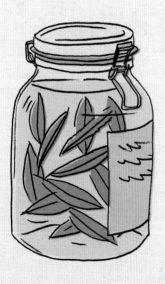

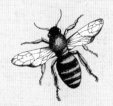

HONEYS AND SYRUPS

The therapeutic qualities of herbs can also be infused into sugar-based preparations, which can preserve them for up to six months and, as Mary Poppins knew, 'a spoonful of sugar helps the medicine go down'. Honey is beneficial in its own right: buy the best affordable quality, preferably local, raw honey. Note that these preparations are inherently calorific and also may not be suitable for diabetics.

To prepare an infused honey: Half-fill a clean jar with the herbs; chop them finely if fresh. Pour over the honey so the herbs are completely submerged. (If the honey is too thick or set to pour, first place its jar in a saucepan and fill the pan until the water is halfway up the side. Heat very gently until the honey is runny.) Fix on the lid and leave for a week to infuse, stirring or shaking daily. Strain out the herbs and repot the infused honey in a clean jar.

To prepare a sugar syrup: Prepare an infusion or decoction (see pages 44–5). Measure the liquid (after straining out the herbs) and pour into a saucepan, adding 10g (2 teaspoons) of unrefined (brown) sugar for every 10ml (2 teaspoons) of liquid. Stir to dissolve the sugar over a low heat, then simmer gently for 10–15 minutes until syrupy but not thick. When cool, pour the syrup into a clean bottle, and label and date it. Once opened, store in the fridge and consume within two months. Dilute to make a hot or cold drink, or take by the teaspoonful.

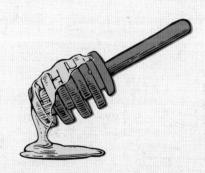

POULTICES AND COMPRESSES

OILS AND VINEGARS

A poultice is the application of herbs directly to the skin to soothe a sting, bite or strain; a compress is similar but uses the infused water not the herbs.

To prepare a poultice: Simmer the fresh herbs in water or vinegar for 5 minutes over a gentle heat. Strain the herbs and place (while still hot) between two pieces of clean muslin cloth or bandages. Wrap or place onto the affected area as soon as the heat is bearable and leave on for an hour.

To prepare a compress: Simmer fresh or dried herbs in water for 5 minutes over a gentle heat. Strain the herbs and use the water to soak a clean facecloth or muslin cloth. Use warm or chilled over the forehead or eyes for a relaxing rest, or wrap onto the affected area for an hour.

Infused oils are made to smooth the skin and to calm or stimulate it, depending on the herbs used. The traditional method of preparation is to leave the herbs and oil in the sun, but it is possible to speed up the process using a bain-marie (see opposite). Infused vinegars, especially when made with raw cider vinegar, are taken by the teaspoonful and can be a prebiotic boost to the immune and digestive systems (see also Fire Cider, page 58). Oxymels, a mix of herbs, sugar and vinegar, are one of the most ancient of herbal preparations.

To prepare an infused oil: After picking fresh herbs, leave them to wilt on a sunny windowsill for one to three days. This removes any excess water that might cause the oil to turn rancid. Alternatively, use freshly dried herbs.

Fill a clean jar with the chosen herbs and pour over the oil, called a carrier oil (olive, almond, jojoba, sunflower or rapeseed are all suitable for this). Ensure the herbs are completely submerged, weighing them down with something glass or ceramic if necessary. Seal the jar and leave on a sunny

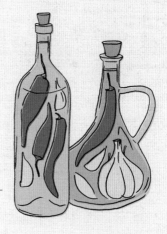

windowsill for four to five weeks, shaking occasionally but ensuring the herbs remain below the surface. The oil is infused once it has changed colour. Different herbs will impart different colours: for example, comfrey will turn the oil green, calendula orange. Strain (without squeezing fresh herbs) into a clean bottle, and label with the contents and date. If the contents separate into water and oil either during infusion or after straining, carefully pour off the oil (and herbs) into a fresh bottle and discard the water. Label and date – the infused oil will keep for six months.

To make infused oil in a bain-marie: Put the herbs and oil into a heatproof bowl set over a pan of barely simmering water. Leave for 2–3 hours, checking the water is still simmering and topping up as necessary. Strain and bottle as above.

To prepare an infused vinegar: Fill a clean jar (with a non-metal lid, as the vinegar will corrode the metal) with herbs and pour over cider vinegar (raw, if possible). Seal and leave to steep for two weeks before straining into a sterilized bottle. Label and date – the vinegar will keep for six months.

To prepare an oxymel: In a large clean jar (with a non-metal lid) mix equal quantities of raw cider vinegar and honey (local and raw, if possible) with two large handfuls of herbs – chop or tear the herbs if they are leafy. To make a runnier oxymel, use more vinegar; for a sweeter taste, add more honey. Almost any herbs can be used, including garlic and berries. Seal and leave for two weeks, shaking daily, then strain into a sterilized jar, label and date. Oxymels will keep for six months and can be taken neat by the teaspoonful, diluted in hot or cold water as a drink, and/or used as a dressing for salads.

Note
Infused oils are distinct from essential oils (which are made by distilling herbs) and are not suitable for culinary use or other consumption.

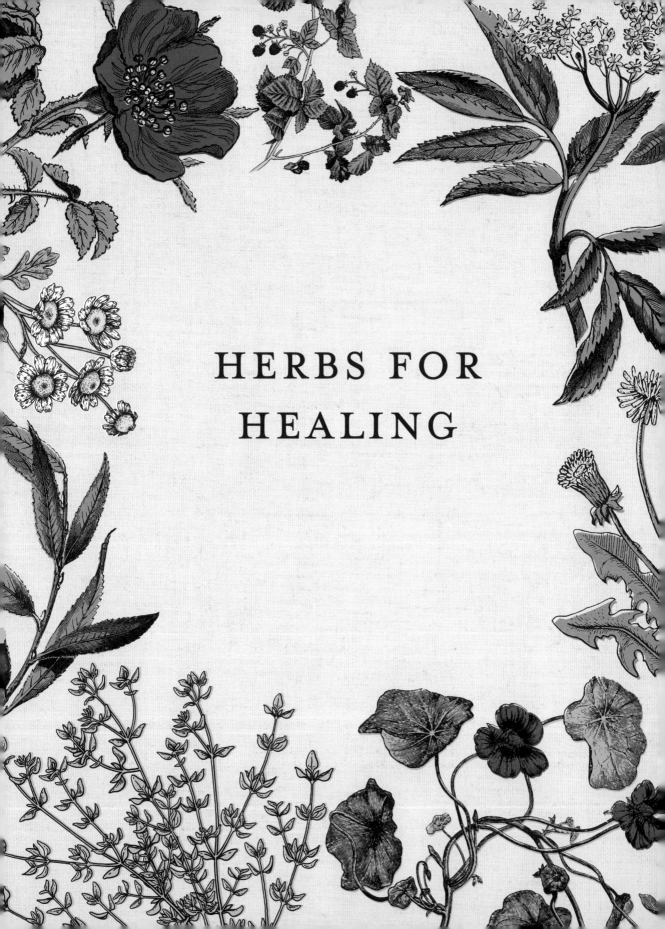

HERBS FOR HEALING

MIND AND MOOD

The human brain is a wondrous thing, capable of so much and still so little understood. For people who live with depression, anxiety or seasonal affective disorder (SAD), or any other condition or situation that can cause a low mood, lethargy, restlessness and lack of sleep, there are herbs that can help to alleviate these symptoms and worries. Fresh air, exercise and mindfulness practice are also incredibly helpful in lowering stress levels and boosting the mood, so getting outside and growing some of these herbs at home could be an all-round good idea. For other helpful herbs for stress and hormonal health, see pages 53 and 60.

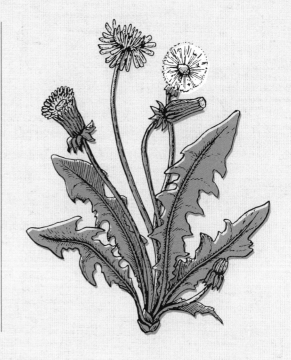

'The lesson I have thoroughly learnt, and wish to pass on to others,
is to know the enduring happiness that the love of a garden gives.'

Gertrude Jekyll, *Wood and Garden* (1899)

HERBS FOR SELF-CARE

When in the grips of a mental health problem, it can be difficult to summon the energy to perform even the simplest of tasks, and so with that in mind, the herbal suggestions here are all in the most basic form: the tisane (see page 44). Invest some time into the ritual of making the tisane to get the most out of the experience.

Make a tisane using a single herb or mix two or more herbs in equal quantities. It could be sweetened with honey, or alternatively infuse the herbs in milk or oat milk and mix with cocoa for a hot chocolate.

To calm frayed nerves: • St John's wort (see page 146) • skullcap (see page 217) • valerian (see page 241) • vervain (see page 242)

To lift the mood: • lemon balm (see page 166) • linden (see page 228) • rose (see page 196)

To give the body and mind a boost: • chilli (see page 100) • chocolate or ginseng (see page 178)

To aid concentration: • ginseng (see page 178) • rosemary (see page 209)

To relax: • chamomile (see page 104) • lavender (see page 156) • linden (see page 228) • passionflower (see page 179) • skullcap (see page 217) • rose (see page 196) • valerian (see page 241)

IMPROVING A LOW LIBIDO

Desire is not something that can be reinstated with a cup of herbal tisane, but using the herbs above to help balance the emotions, coupled with fresh air and exercise, may go some way towards improving a low libido. Otherwise, ashwagandha (see page 245), cardamom (see page 126) and ginseng (see page 178) are all reputed aphrodisiacs.

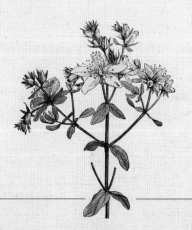

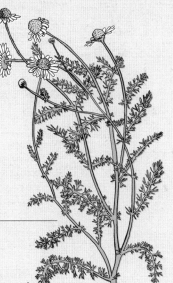

STRESS, IMMUNITY AND BALANCE

Using herbal remedies at home is largely about supporting overall health and maintaining a strong and balanced body and mind, with some treatment of symptoms of illness and injury. Getting a good night's sleep is a crucial part of feeling well, and there are various herbs that can help with this and also with increasing the body's ability to resist stresses.

ADAPTING TO CHANGE

Adaptogens are compounds that assist the body in adapting to change, for example withstanding intense or prolonged periods of external stress, and increasing its resistance to illness. Herbal adaptogens include ginseng (see page 178), ashwagandha (see page 245), liquorice (see page 140) and astragalus (see page 90).

HAVING A GOOD NIGHT'S SLEEP

A tisane or bath using one or more of these herbs can help the body relax and drift off into a restful sleep:
• ashwagandha (see page 245)
• Californian poppy (see page 128)

• chamomile (see page 104)
• lavender (see page 156)
• lemon balm (see page 166)
• linden (see page 228)
• passionflower (see page 179)
• valerian (see page 241)

HERBAL IMMUNITY BOOSTERS

In late summer and early autumn, hedgerows and gardens are full of natural sources of vitamin C and immune-boosting compounds, such as elderberry, rosehips and hawthorn berries. Make a batch or two of syrups (see pages 197 and 213) to drink, diluted, in hot water through the autumn and winter to stave off the cold and flu season. Other good herbs to boost the immune system are echinacea (see page 124) and bilberries (see page 240). Make them into tinctures and jam respectively.

Alternatively, make an oxymel or a simple infused vinegar with a mixture of fresh or dried berries such as elderberries, rosehips, hawthorn berries or bilberries and take daily (1-2 tablespoonsful of infused vinegar can be diluted in a little hot water and take before breakfast).

COLDS AND FLU

Preventative measures are not infallible, and where there is a need to relieve symptoms of colds and flus, such as sore throats, headaches and congestion, herbs can assist and support the body's own defences so that it can rid itself of the infection.

HELPFUL HERBAL DRINKS

Any herbal drink will bring comfort and hydration – both essential when in the grips of a nasty cold – and hot tisanes and cordials will also help to warm the hands around the mug. A cup of chamomile and/or elderflower and linden tisane before bed can help induce drowsiness when sleeping is difficult. Rosehip or elderberry syrups (see pages 197 and 213 for recipes), diluted in hot water, will continue to support the immune system, and eating plenty of garlic, ginger and nettles will similarly boost the body's immunity and give it plenty of nutrition. Meadowsweet cordial (see page 133) diluted with cold water for a refreshing drink can also provide some pain relief from headaches.

STEAMING

Steaming is an excellent way of clearing a blocked nose and stuffy head. Fill a bowl with boiling water and a handful of herbs such as eucalyptus, mint, sage, lemon balm and thyme, lean over and inhale the fragrant steam in through the nose and out through the mouth. Covering the head and bowl with a towel helps to keep the steam and volatile oils around you, and stay under for as long as you can bear!

Making a hot foot bath in a similar way and adding 1–2 teaspoons of mustard powder, to warm the feet, will stimulate the circulation.

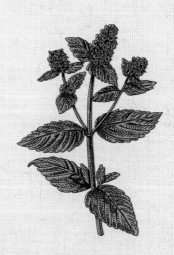

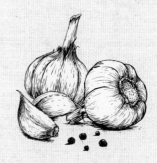

SAGE GARGLE

A tincture of sage (see page 206) will help soothe a sore throat and act as an antiseptic – add cloves (see page 222) for extra antiseptic and anaesthetic qualities. Dilute 1 tablespoon of tincture in around 150–250ml (½–1 cup) of boiled, and then cooled to lukewarm, water and gargle. Swallow or spit – it's not the tastiest.

For immediate relief when the cupboard is bare, try making a sage hot-water infusion of double strength and allow it to cool to lukewarm before gargling. See also page 125 for an echinacea and sage gargle.

GARLIC HONEY AND ONION SYRUP

Both raw garlic and onions (see page 74) are considered herbs and are effective, if pungent, for congestion, phlegm and coughs. Mixing them with sugar preserves them, makes them more palatable and creates an unctuous syrup which coats the throat to bring relief. Take a teaspoonful of either up to six times a day for symptomatic relief, or once a day as a preventative measure.

To make garlic honey: Peel and finely slice the cloves of three bulbs/heads of garlic and put into a sterilized jar. Cover with honey, stirring to ensure all the garlic is covered. Seal, label and date, and leave to infuse. It will be ready the next day. Use within three months.

To make onion syrup: Peel and finely slice an onion into rings. Layer the rings in a sterilized jar, alternating with layers of sugar (any type is fine). Seal, label and date, and leave overnight – the sugar will almost dissolve the onion, creating a syrup. Strain out any remaining onion after 24 hours and use the syrup within 4–5 days. Store in the refrigerator.

THE DIGESTIVE SYSTEM

The gut and its myriad complexities are still relatively little understood by medical science, but anyone who has ever suffered a digestive complaint will know that an unhappy digestion can affect one's entire being. Indeed, it is now thought that the gut biome – the collective name for the trillions of bacteria and fungi that inhabit the digestive tract – is something akin to a second brain, such is its effect on mood, immunity or lack thereof, metabolism and body weight.

There are many helpful herbs that will support a healthy working digestion when used regularly. Those listed below are all easy to incorporate into the diet in the form of tisanes.

For indigestion, constipation, bloating and flatulence:

· angelica (see page 84)

· chamomile (see page 104)

· fennel (see page 134)

· peppermint (see page 168) – avoid with acid reflux

· plantain seed (see page 188) – for constipation, mix with other foods

For after diarrhoea and to restore nutrient levels:

· blackberry, fruit and leaf (see page 200)

· chamomile (see page 104)

· nettle (see page 237)

· thyme (see page 227)

For nausea:

· angelica (see page 84)

· cardamom (see page 126)

· ginger (see page 246)

...plus all the herbs listed for indigestion.

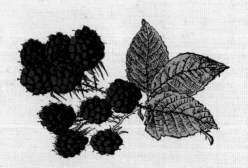

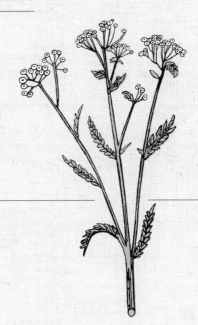

BITTER HERBS

Over time, many vegetables have had their bitterness bred out of them to please our palates, which naturally prefer sweeter tastes. However, bitterness in foods also signals the presence of beneficial compounds that aid digestion and the absorption of nutrients from our food, as well as supporting liver function, which, in turn, helps the body to eliminate toxins. Bitter herbs have been known to be good for us for so long that they make several appearances in the Bible, usually in a similar vein to this passage from Numbers 9:11 '…eat it with unleavened bread and bitter herbs.'

Brassicas such as kale, cabbage and Brussels sprouts are all good sources of bitter compounds, as are coffee, bitter citrus fruits such as grapefruit, chicory, endive, wild rocket (arugula) and chocolate with a high percentage of cocoa (85 per cent or more).

The pre-dinner drink, the aperitif, is also traditionally bitter to help with digestion: add bitters to a cocktail, or make a tincture with one or more of the bitter herbs below and take a scant teaspoonful mixed with 2 tablespoons of water 15–30 minutes before dining.

- angelica, root (see page 84)
- burdock, root/seeds (see page 86)
- chamomile, flower (see page 104)
- chicory, root (see page 106)
- dandelion, root/leaf (see page 226)
- ginger, root (see page 246)
- yarrow, leaf/flower (see page 68)

Note
Bitter herbs should be avoided during pregnancy and in cases of gastric ulcers.

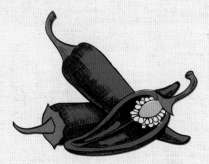

FIRE CIDER

As the name suggests, this recipe is spicy! Raw cider vinegar is infused with herbs and taken either daily or when required to alleviate symptoms. Although fire cider will stimulate the digestion, it is also helpful in a number of other complaints, especially sore throats, coughs and colds. The exact proportions are not crucial – every herbalist has their own version – and the recipe can be adapted to taste and according to the availability of ingredients.

1 (red) onion

2 heads/bulbs of garlic

3–5 fresh chillies (red or green)

1 unwaxed lemon

10cm (4in) piece of fresh turmeric root

10cm (4in) piece of fresh ginger root

5cm (2in) piece of fresh horseradish root

2 tsp black peppercorns , crushed

a handful of fresh sprigs of rosemary, sage and thyme

1 litre (4 cups) raw cider vinegar

Peel and slice the onion and garlic. Finely slice the chillies and lemon, and finely slice or grate the turmeric, ginger and horseradish.

Layer these ingredients with the peppercorns and herb sprigs into a wide-necked sterilized large jar (with a plastic or rubber seal, not metal, which the vinegar could corrode).

Cover with the vinegar, giving it a shake to ensure there is no air trapped under the surface.

Seal and leave to infuse in a cool, dark place for two to four weeks, shaking the jar gently every day or so.

Strain into a clean sterilized bottle, label and date (it will keep for a year).

Take 1–2 tablespoons daily, mixed with a little water, if liked, before food.

For sore throats, mix with honey (and water) and gargle or swallow.

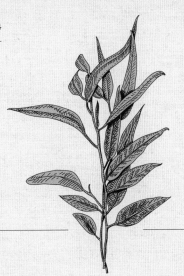

ACHES AND PAINS

At its most basic, a herbal approach to treating minor injuries is as simple as crushing a plantain leaf and rubbing the juice over a nettle sting. Herbs can both help with the relief of chronic conditions such as arthritis and with short-term injuries such as sprains.

TIGHT MUSCLES

A bath, using some or all the herbs listed below, is a relaxing way to soothe tiredness and aches. Add Epsom salts, if desired.
Comfrey (see page 221)
Eucalyptus (see page 131)
Lavender (see page 156)
Meadowsweet (see page 132)
Rosemary (see page 209)

JOINT PAIN

Incorporating turmeric, chilli and black pepper into the diet helps to stimulate the circulation and reduce inflammation, easing any pain. Infusions or tinctures of rosemary, St John's wort and cramp bark can provide relief, while meadowsweet, a natural painkiller, can be taken in a cordial (see page 133).

Herbs high in antioxidants with cleansing properties, such as rosehip, nettle, cleavers and dandelion, can also help to limit inflammation.

FIRST-AID POULTICES

Follow the directions on page 48 to make a poultice or compress. Sage leaves (see page 206) can be efficacious for a sprain or strain, as can comfrey (see page 221).

CRAMPS AND PAINFUL MUSCLES

Painful aches and cramps, including period pains, can be alleviated by a slow massage of herbal oil into the affected area. The act of massaging and the herbs in the oil both stimulate the circulation and relax the muscles, which can relieve pain and cramping.

Make an infused oil (see page 48) of equal parts ginger root (see page 246) and rosemary leaves (see page 209). Add 2 teaspoons of black peppercorns (see page 186) or 1 chilli pepper (see page 100) per 100ml (3½fl oz) of oil for an even more invigorating mix. Wash hands thoroughly after using the infused oil and avoid contact with the eyes, genital area and sensitive skin.

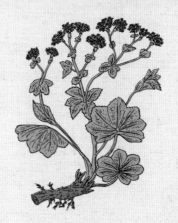

WOMEN'S HEALTH

No two women are the same, and neither are their monthly cycles or responses to their hormones, nor the rollercoaster of hormonal symptoms that can typify the perimenopause and menopause. Learning to work with, not against, those hormones can be a huge first step in empowering women to take control of their own bodies and health, and it is as simple as noting down mood and physical symptoms in a diary for a few months and comparing them to the stage of the menstrual cycle. Herbs can be a helpful support for overall health and hormonal balance, as well as useful, gentle solutions to symptoms such as period pain (see page 59).

HELPFUL HERBS FOR WOMEN

· cramp bark (see page 243)
· ginger (see page 246)
· lady's mantle (see page 72)
· lemon balm (see page 166)
· nettle (see page 237)
· raspberry leaf (see page 200)
· rose (see page 196)
· selfheal (see page 191)
· yarrow (see page 68)

Tisanes of lady's mantle, raspberry leaf and nettle can support overall reproductive health. Nettle, yarrow and selfheal are useful for heavy menstrual bleeding or during the menopause to boost mineral levels and promote healing. Lady's mantle, rose and lemon balm can help to balance the hormones and boost low moods. All of these herbs can be taken as hot-water infusions, either singly or combined. A tincture of cramp bark can be effective against period pain, and ginger in any form reduces nausea.

BALANCING ACT TEA

Equal quantities of dried lady's mantle, linden flowers and rose flowers, mixed and stored in a pretty tin, will make a calming, restorative tea to balance the hormones at any time of the month or to ease menopausal symptoms. A cupful can be drunk up to three times a day. Take time over the process of making and drinking the tea to give a little mindful moment of peace.

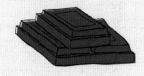

FIERY TRUFFLES

This recipe combines high-percentage cocoa chocolate, which is full of both antioxidants and mood-boosting compounds, with naturally sweet and fibre-rich dates, to make tasty truffles that are a healthier treat to meet chocolate cravings and mood swings. This basic recipe could be adapted to increase, reduce or omit the chilli, according to taste, and/or include 1 tablespoon of chopped dried herbs such as nettle (for iron replacement) or rose, plantain seeds or lady's mantle (for hormone balancing). The truffles are also delicious with the addition of chopped nuts, chopped crystallized ginger and/or dried cranberries, but experiment with your favourite flavours.

100g (3½oz) dark chocolate (85 per cent cocoa solids)
seeds fromv1 vanilla pod or 1 tsp vanilla extract
150g (²⁄₃cup) stoned dates
1 small dried red chilli or small pinch of chilli flakes

1 tbsp raw honey
½ tsp ground cinnamon
1 tbsp chopped dried herbs (optional)
1–2 tbsp chopped nuts or dried fruit (optional)
cocoa powder, for dusting

Break the chocolate into a bowl and set it over a small pan of barely simmering water to melt.

Put the vanilla seeds or extract, dates, chilli, honey, cinnamon and dried herbs (if using) in a food processor and blitz to a paste.

Take the melted chocolate off the heat and stir in the date paste until combined. Stir in the chopped nuts/fruit (if using), then refrigerate until it is cool enough to scoop and roll into balls. Roll teaspoonsful of the mix into a ball, then roll in cocoa powder. Store in the fridge for up to two weeks and eat no more than 4 per day.

Note
A number of herbs are not advised during pregnancy, breastfeeding or attempts to conceive. Please exercise caution and consult a medical practitioner and herbalist before using any herbal remedies in these situations.

CHILDREN'S HEALTH

Although the use of home remedies for children should rightly be treated with caution (see below), there are many herbal options, many of which have been used for centuries, that are soothing, gentle and effective ways to support a child who is under the weather or in need of a little extra care and attention. From a chamomile infusion for an upset tummy, famously dispensed to Peter Rabbit after he gorged himself in Mr McGregor's garden, to a honey-sweetened tisane of equal parts calming elderflowers and linden flowers to help them get off to sleep, herbs can be part of the everyday diet of children as well as adults, and set them up for a lifetime of turning to nature to heal themselves.

HELPFUL HERBS

Chamomile (see page 104)
Elderflower (see page 210)
Linden flower (see page 228)
Marigold (see page 96)

Infused honeys are a wonderfully easy way to tempt children into taking a herbal remedy. Have a jar of linden flowers and elderflower, or lemon balm-infused honey to hand to help calm them when they are anxious. Elderberry syrup, diluted in hot water, can help boost their immune systems to fight school's never-ending onslaught of cough and cold germs, and no child can resist the gooey temptation of snapping off a piece of aloe vera leaf to squeeze out the

Note
It is not advised to give herbal preparations to any child under the age of two, and when considering giving internal herbal preparations to children under the age of 14, always dilute the dose and test with just a small volume first. Children aged two to six can be given up to 30 per cent of an adult dose; children aged six to ten up to 50 per cent of an adult dose; and children aged 10–14 up to 80 per cent of an adult dose. Always patch-test external remedies on an adult first and then on the child. Some herbs are not suitable for children in any form; check the contraindications for individual herbs.

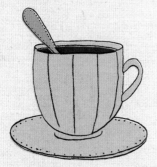

gel onto a bite or burn. In summer, use a lolly mould to freeze infusions such as mint and chamomile, or elderflower and lemon balm (sweetened with a spoonful of honey, if liked) into lollies to calm tummy aches and frayed nerves.

BEDTIME COCOA

Hot chocolate plays a part in the Chelsea Physic Garden's history, and this recipe uses herb-infused honeys to calm and relax children in the evening. Use oat milk rather than cow's milk for a dairy-free alternative and one that adds to the sleep-inducing effect – oats contain relaxing compounds such as melatonin.

Gently heat a small mugful of milk in a saucepan (add a cinnamon stick and/or vanilla pod, if liked and simmer over a low heat for 5–10 minutes). Put 1 tbsp cocoa powder into the child's favourite mug, pour in a splash of the hot milk and stir to make a paste. Strain out the cinnamon and vanilla, then pour the rest of the milk into the mug, stirring or whisking constantly. Stir in linden flower- or chamomile-infused honey to taste, then serve.

SKIN-CALMING BALM

This soothing balm, suitable for adults and children alike, calms irritated skin and rashes. Use it on nappy rash, chapped skin around the nose and mouth or any other patches of dry skin.

8 dried calendula flower heads or 8 tsp dried calendula petals
40g (3 tbsp) shea or cocoa butter
60ml (¼ cup) jojoba or olive oil
4 tsp beeswax
5–10 drops of lavender essential oil (optional)

Put the petals, butter and oil in a heatproof bowl, set over a small pan of simmering water. Stir and leave to infuse for 2–3 hours (check the water level periodically and top up if necessary).
Strain out the petals then return the mixture to the bowl and add the beeswax, stirring gently to dissolve.
Remove from the heat and cool slightly before whisking in the essential oil, if using. Pour into cans, tubs or jars and label and date. Apply a small quantity to the affected skin as needed, and use within one year.

SKIN AND HAIR

A number of herbs are used on the skin for their astringent (pore-tightening) qualities. Here, perhaps more so than with other home remedies, the fragrance of the herbs helps to make the preparations feel luxurious and relaxing. Taking such bitter herbs as cleavers, dandelion, chicory root, dock and angelica internally, either as a tisane or added to food, can help to cleanse the body of impurities that can cause skin problems.

HELPFUL HERBS

• cleavers (see page 135) – for general skin health and brightness
• chamomile (see page 104) – especially for sensitive skin
• echinacea (see page 124) – a study showed a tincture was effective for acne
• elderflower (see page 210) – for brightening the skin tone
• lady's mantle (see page 72) – for mature skin
• marigold (see page 96) – to soothe skin irritation
• rose (see page 196) – for mature skin
• rosemary (see page 209) – for the hair/scalp
• witch hazel (see page 142) – to cool and tighten the skin

ROSEMARY HAIR TONIC

Rosemary is especially good at stimulating the scalp, and can promote a healthy, flake-free scalp and strong shiny hair growth. Thyme or sage leaves, both of which have cleansing properties, can also be added. Sage will also darken the hair a shade or two. Make this tonic as needed, store in a sterilized bottle in the fridge – use it within a week.

6 tbsp fresh (or 3 tbsp dried) rosemary leaves
6 tbsp fresh (or 3 tbsp dried) sage or thyme leaves (optional)
1 litre (4 cups) boiling water
3 tbsp cider vinegar

Put the herbs into a saucepan or jug, pour over the water, cover and leave until cool. Strain out the herbs and stir in the vinegar. To use, pour or spray a third of the mix over the hair as a final rinse after washing and conditioning, massaging it into the scalp well. There is no need to rinse it out.

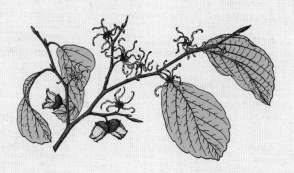

WITCH HAZEL TONER/AFTERSHAVE

Witch hazel helps to tighten the pores and reduce inflammation after washing or shaving. Both the stems and the leaves are used for this toner, so it is prepared as both a decoction and an infusion. Store in sterilized bottles for up to six months, switching to a spray bottle top when you come to use it. Leaves can be dried to use with twigs to make supplies all year round.

50g (2oz) young witch hazel branches or dried leaves
*   and bark*
300ml (1¼ cups) cold water
50ml (¼ cup) vodka or rum (at least 40 per cent
*   ABV/80 per cent proof)*

Remove the leaves from the branches and set aside. Chop the branches into small pieces and put into a saucepan with the water. Cover and bring to the boil, then simmer for an hour. Take the pan off the heat, stir in the leaves and alcohol, cover again and leave to infuse overnight. Strain into sterilized bottles, label and date.

HAND AND BODY SCRUB

An infused sugar-based scrub is an easy way to incorporate healing herbs into a beauty regimen, and jars of the infused sugars make lovely gifts, especially when they have been personalized to suit the skin and favourite scents of the recipient.

For an exfoliating scrub for dry skin, mix chopped dried herbs into a jar of granulated sugar – try lavender, rose petals, lemon verbena, lemon balm or mallow – and store until needed. To use, simply pour a small quantity into the hands and rub gently into the skin, rinsing with warm water.

A softer alternative uses brown sugar (any type) mixed with herb-infused oil. Simply mix 25ml (1½ tbsp) herb-infused oil per 100g (½ cup) of brown sugar, adding up to 20 drops of essential oil if desired. Use in the same way as above.

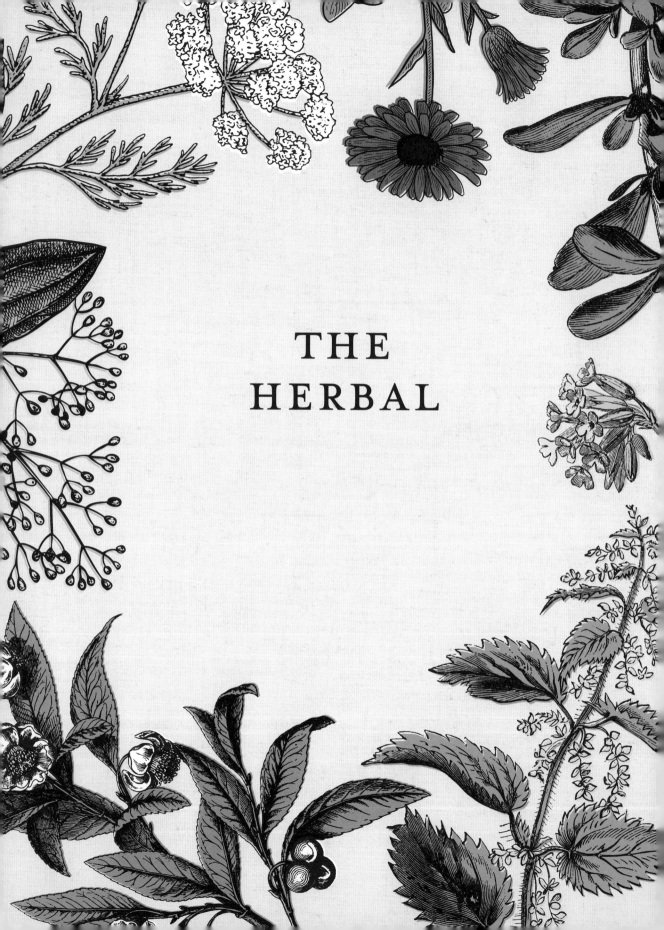

THE
HERBAL

A HERBAL GUIDE

A plant that can adapt to many different growing situations and a changing climate will persist down the generations – and mankind will likely find a use for it. Nettles (see page 237) are a prime example of a relatively invasive herb that has been allowed to commandeer our hedgerows and wild fields because of its myriad therapeutic, culinary and other uses. This symbiotic relationship between mankind and semi-cultivated plants is known as crypto-cropping. Other herbs need more careful cultivation and preservation, and while some have been overexploited in the wild and are now endangered, others such as garlic have been heavily used for so long that a truly wild species no longer exists.

Herbs are still a part of our lives, whether in our gardens or our over-the-counter medicines. The herbs included here are but a small selection of the many thousands of useful plants grown in the Chelsea Physic Garden and worldwide. They are the herbs best known for having some therapeutic benefit or that have made significant contributions to the history of medicine. Most are also easily accessible for preparing simple healing home remedies, mainly because they are common garden or hedgerow plants.

This herbal is intended as an interesting guide to the plants in the Chelsea Physic Garden (and your garden). Perhaps, too, it will be an inspiring starting point for understanding more about the healing power of nature, and how herbs can add variety, seasonality and richness to a healthy, balanced lifestyle.

ACHILLEA MILLEFOLIUM

Yarrow *Soldier's woundwort, milfoil, staunchweed*

This aromatic herb has a long history of being used internally and externally
for a wide range of complaints. The white flowers are often seen gracing
verges and hedgerows. For preparations it is best to use the species, but
'Lilac Beauty', grown at the Garden, is an attractive ornamental cultivar.
When added to compost, yarrow will accelerate its decomposition.

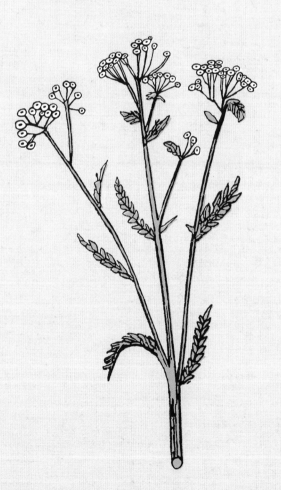

Caution
Extended or heavy use can cause skin rashes
and increased skin sensitivity to light; the
aerial parts of the plant can be phytotoxic.
Yarrow is a member of the Asteraceae family
and should be avoided by anyone with
allergies to these plants. Contraindicated
during pregnancy.

Cultivation
Yarrow prefers well-drained soil in full sun, but
can grow more or less anywhere. A herbaceous
perennial, it forms a fully hardy mat of feathery
leaves at the base, with flower stems rising to
a height of around 50cm (20in). Yarrow is an
excellent attractor of beneficial insects, such as
hoverflies, to the garden.

A History of Healing

Yarrow's Latin genus name, *Achillea*, is from Achilles, the Greek warrior of the eponymous heel, which refers to the plant's long use in staunching the blood flow of and imparting an antibacterial effect onto a wound. Parkinson recommended an oil of yarrow to 'stayeth the shedding of the haire'. Before the introduction of hops, yarrow was used to add flavour to beer in medieval Europe.

Other species of yarrow are also bitter and aromatic. Musk yarrow (*A. erba-rotta* subsp. *moschata*) is used in perfumery and the making of alcoholic drinks, including the liqueur iva; sneezewort (*A. ptarmica*) was historically used for snuff; the sweetly perfumed English mace (*A. ageratum*) can be used as a herbal flavouring in the kitchen but was traditionally used as a strewing herb, scattered across the floor, so as to release its scent when walked upon.

To divine success in a romantic relationship, a yarrow leaf was traditionally used to tickle the nostrils while reciting 'Yarroway, Yarroway, bear a white blow; If my love love me my nose will bleed now.' Given yarrow's use in staunching rather than stimulating blood flow, this was perhaps a trick employed by mothers to dissuade their daughters from an inappropriate match!

The most significant constituent to have been isolated from the herb is the anti-inflammatory and anti-allergenic compound azulene.

Harvesting

Flowers are dried before using, so cut the stems of the flower stalks at the base in summer. They should be fully in flower but newly opened, so avoid those that have been in flower for a few weeks. Cut only as much as is needed, leaving the rest for the insects. The leaves can be picked through the spring and summer.

How to Use

The flowers (dried or fresh) can be made into a tisane, tincture, infused syrup or honey and are helpful in easing the symptoms of indigestion, strengthening the circulation, lowering high blood pressure, relieving varicose veins and haemorrhoids and regulating menstrual flow (see also page 60). The leaves can be infused in a tincture with the flowers or eaten raw in salads. As a herbal bitter, yarrow has a beneficial effect on digestion.

Yarrow leaves can be crushed and applied directly to the skin or used as a poultice to staunch the bleeding of wounds or nosebleeds (as a small plug for the base of the nostrils). The essential oil added to balms and other external creams or an infused oil made with yarrow can be applied to skin injuries and complaints, such as eczema, where it has an antimicrobial and anti-inflammatory effect.

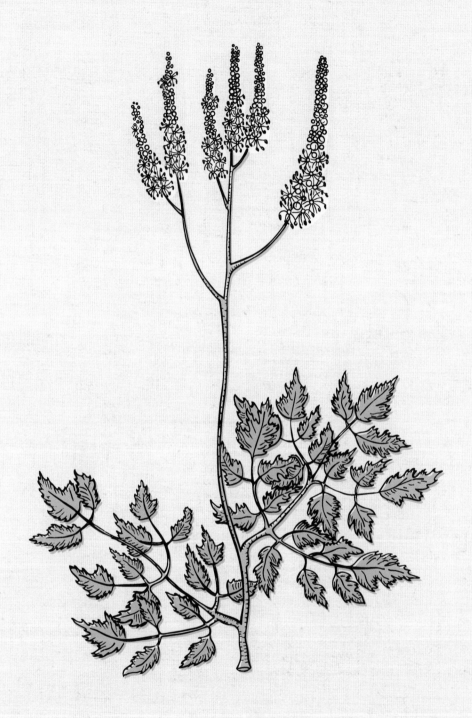

ACTAEA RACEMOSA (SYN. CIMICIFUGA RACEMOSA)

Black cohosh *Squaw root, black snakeroot*

Black cohosh has attractive but malodorous spikes of white flowers in summer. Relatives of the plant are used in ornamental gardens for their attractive appearance.

Caution
Contraindicated in pregnancy; some countries restrict its growth and/or use. Consult a medical professional before taking black cohosh if you have a liver condition and/or have been diagnosed with cancer, especially breast cancer.

Cultivation
Black cohosh prefers a moist, rich soil in partial or dappled shade. A fully hardy herbaceous perennial, it can reach up to 2m (6½ft) tall when in flower, and has a spread of around 60cm (2ft). Cut back old growth in late winter and mulch annually.

A History of Healing
Traditionally used in Native American medicine for menstrual problems and to alleviate the symptoms of the menopause, black cohosh has been found to be effective for the treatment of the latter in modern clinical trials, especially when combined with St John's wort.

It is suggested that it stimulates the brain to produce more oestrogen, which can also help reduce the incidence of osteoporosis during and after the menopause. It is also anti-inflammatory and used in the traditional treatment of rheumatoid arthritis.

Harvesting
Dig up a portion of the roots in autumn and use fresh or dry to store.

How to Use
A tincture prepared with the fresh or dried roots or a decoction of the dried roots can be taken for menstrual and postpartum pains, to relieve menopausal symptoms and for bronchial complaints. Tablets made from the powdered root are available from herbal suppliers but they should be taken with caution and never to excess.

ORIGINS
Northwest and
central Europe,
Greece

ALCHEMILLA VULGARIS

Lady's mantle *Lion's foot*

The tiny hairs on the leaves of these plants hold rain and dew droplets so beautifully that the plant was thought magical – it has been suggested that *Alchemilla* derives from 'alchemy', the magical art of turning base metals into gold. Several plants are known as lady's mantle: *A. vulgaris*, which has a synonym of *A. xanthochlora*, and *A. mollis*, which is widely known as an ornamental garden and cut flower plant. *A. alpina*, the smaller alpine version, has slightly different herbal medicine applications and is reputedly more potent, but for the most part all lady's mantle species can be used interchangeably.

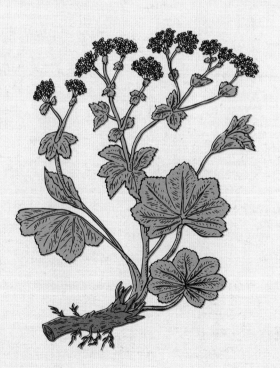

Caution
Contraindicated during pregnancy and periods of constipation.

Cultivation
Fully hardy, lady's mantle is a herbaceous perennial that forms a low clump of soft leaves, from which floppy stems of acid green flowers rise in late spring until early autumn. It reaches only 50cm (20in) in height and breadth, but spreads easily by seed if the flowers are not cut back once they start to brown. It will grow in most situations, but prefers moist but well-drained soil in dappled shade or full sun and will not grow well on lime soils. If more than one named species is grown in a garden, self-sown seedlings should be treated as hybrids. The alpine lady's mantle will grow well in pots or window boxes, and reaches around 20cm (8in) in height and spread.

A History of Healing

Lady's mantle is astringent and used to staunch the flow of blood from wounds, often combined with yarrow (see page 68). Parkinson wrote that it 'is accounted as one of the most singular wound herbes that is', suggesting that the wound should be externally dressed with the leaves and a decoction of them drunk as well.

However, as its folk name suggests, it has also long been prized as useful in treating all manner of complaints particular to women, notably menstrual irregularity, heavy menstrual flow and menopausal symptoms. It was said to tone the womb and make it more receptive to conception, as well as reputedly tightening the genitals, to the extent that Andres de Laguna's 1570 translation of *De Materia Medica* by Dioscorides reported that alchemilla is 'a thousand times sold' to those women who desired to appear to be a virgin. For those women perhaps more advanced in years, it was apparently more useful in contracting the breast tissue: Parkinson wrote that 'it helpeth also such maides or women that have overgreat flagging breasts, causing them to grow lesse and hard, being both drunke, and outwardly applyed'.

Harvesting

Both the flowers and leaves can be used, although the flowers also make a pretty cut flower mixed in a posy. Cut off all the fresh flowers and leaves (drying and storing those that can't be used fresh) and the plant will regrow new leaves and possibly flowers in the same season, allowing for a second harvest.

How to Use

Add fresh or dried flowers or leaves to tisanes to aid menstrual regularity and to relieve period pains (see also page 60) – it is best drunk daily for this. Once cooled, a hot-water infusion can also be used as an external vaginal wash to ease the symptoms of infections such as thrush.

To harness the astringent properties of lady's mantle, boil the flowers or leaves in a saucepan of water for 3–5 minutes and strain. The resulting infusion can be drunk as a tea to alleviate diarrhoea, or applied as a toner for oily or spotty skin.

ALLIUM

Garlic and onion

For each of the plants detailed in his herbal, Culpeper first gave a description or said merely that the plant was so well known it didn't need one. Under garlic, he simply wrote that the 'offensiveness of the breath' of someone who has eaten garlic was so potent that, like a bloodhound set on a trail, it 'will lead you by the nose to the knowledge thereof, and direct you to the place where it grows in gardens'.

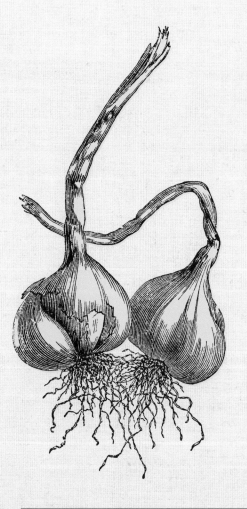

Both garlic and onions belong to the large Alliaceae family, known as alliums, which also includes wild garlic (ransoms), leeks, chives and the ornamental allium flower bulbs. Garlic probably originated in central Asia but has been cultivated for so long that the species is not actually found in the wild – the *sativum* part of its name, meaning 'cultivated', denotes this – and

GARLIC BREATH

The 'offensiveness of the breath' mentioned by Culpeper (see above) is caused by the sulphurous compounds in the garlic cloves, but take heart that it is these very compounds that are bringing the health benefits. Of course, as the French saying goes, if everyone was always eating garlic, there wouldn't be a problem. However, assuming that is not the case, chewing parsley or any plant with an aniseed taste, such as fennel or liquorice, can help to neutralize the issue.

there are records of its use even five thousand years ago in Babylonia. All the *Allium sativum* varieties can be used interchangeably. Other types of garlic, such as elephant garlic, with its enormous, less pungent cloves, are actually different species. While beneficial, they are not as potent.

Caution

Those with blood-clotting disorders or those taking anticoagulants should consult a medical professional before dramatically increasing the quantity of garlic in their diet.

Cultivation

Garlic is hardy and should be planted in the autumn using bulbs grown specifically for planting. Break them apart and plant the cloves in well-drained soil in a sunny position. They will be ready to harvest in early summer once the single cloves have grown into a full bulb. The flower stalks (scapes) and flowers can be eaten either green (fresh) or dried, to store, as can the bulbs. Onions prefer similar conditions: plant sets or sow seed in spring.

A History of Healing

Garlic has been vital to civilization over the millennia. It was found in Tutankhamun's tomb, and was famously given daily to slaves building the pyramids to keep them in good health. Pliny the Elder listed garlic as a medicine for 60 different ailments and, as recently as the early 20th century, it was used as a treatment for tuberculosis, typhoid and as a wound dressing. Onions have a similar history. Both are used the world over in cuisine and herbal medicine,

although Buddhists avoid alliums as they consider them too stimulating to the body to be compatible with meditation. The skins of onions are also a natural dye of earthy coloured tones.

The bubonic plague pandemic in medieval Europe was an opportunity for many herbal preparations to be tested but also for much quackery: a bunch of onions hanging on the door is less likely to have warded off the plague than actually eating them. One of the traditional remedies from this period is Four Thieves Vinegar. Legend has it that the thieves were robbing plague victims and yet not succumbing to the disease themselves. In return for a more lenient sentence, they revealed the secret of their immunity: dousing themselves with a vinegar infused with herbs variously listed as sage, thyme, rosemary, lavender, juniper and garlic, which certainly would have deterred the fleas now known to transmit the disease.

Modern trials have proven garlic's specific effectiveness in lowering blood pressure and cholesterol levels. It also has a beneficial effect on blood sugar levels and is known to have antibiotic qualities. When a thousand-year-old recipe for a garlic preparation from *Bald's Leechbook* (an English collection of herbal preparation recipes dating from *c.*950 CE) was tested against a superbug resistant to most modern antibiotic drugs, 90 per cent of the bacteria were killed.

Garlic in Myths and Legends

Inevitably, for a plant so long used as food and medicine, a number of legends have grown up around it. Garlic has long been associated with evil-doing; it was said that when Satan left the Garden of Eden after tempting Eve to eat the apple, garlic and onion plants sprang up in his footsteps. Generally, though, garlic is used to ward off evil, notably vampires, but also witches and other evil spirits. Perhaps because of its pungent nature, William Coles in his herbal *The Art of Simpling* (1656) suggests that putting garlic into the soil will cause moles to 'leap out of the ground presently'. This seems unlikely, but garlic is widely used today by domestic organic growers as an infused water spray to deter bugs such as aphids from their crops. Chewing garlic was considered to give physical advantages, too: Roman soldiers ate it before going into battle, as did athletes before racing – allegedly, it would prevent one's competitors getting ahead.

How to Use

Garlic and onions are safe to use and yet powerfully effective for a number of health complaints, notably colds and flu. Adding onions and especially garlic to the diet or taking them regularly as preparations can also benefit the circulation and heart health as well as overall immunity and the digestion (alliums contain inulin, a prebiotic that promotes healthy gut flora).

Garlic and onions are most effective when used raw, and garlic is more beneficial crushed rather than sliced. To allow the helpful compounds of allicin to develop, leave the crushed/chopped garlic and onions for 5–10 minutes before eating, or infuse them in preparations such as Garlic Honey, Onion Syrup and Fire Cider (see pages 55 and 58). Take daily, and especially in the case of chest infections, colds, flu and other such bronchial complaints.

MAKING A GARLIC OR ONION PLAIT

This traditional way of storing alliums is also convenient and practical. It keeps the bulbs dry, and hanging them at a kitchen window means that they will always be to hand. Softneck varieties have the long, floppy leaves needed to weave together the bulbs in a plait; hardneck varieties can be tied together in bunches.

Collect together the dried bulbs in late summer, once there is no moisture left in the upper leaves. Brush off any remaining soil and cut off the dangly roots. Start the plait with three bulbs, with a larger bulb in the centre. Complete one full turn of braiding (right stem over the centre one, so the right becomes the centre; left stem over the new centre one) before adding in the next bulb and plaiting it in, adding to the centre, right then left in turn. Always put the larger bulbs in the centre and the smaller ones on the side and braid each one in before adding a new one. Once all the bulbs have been used up, braid the stems for a few more turns, tie them together and hang in a cool, dry place.

ALOE VERA (SYN. *ALOE BARBADENSIS*)

Aloe *Barbados aloe*

Aloe makes a good house plant, perfect for the kitchen windowsill, where its stems can be easily snapped off and applied to burns sustained while cooking.

Caution
Do not take internally without consulting a medical professional and especially not in cases of pregnancy, breastfeeding, haemorrhoids or kidney disease.

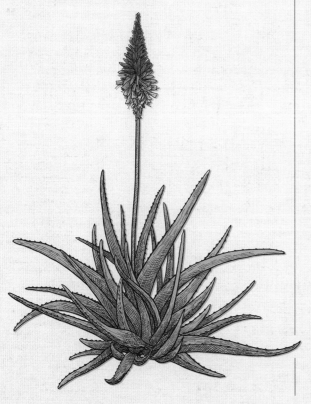

Cultivation
A tender succulent, aloe requires a very well-drained soil and a bright position. It will reach around 60cm (2ft) in height and spread.

A History of Healing
There is evidence of aloe being used as far back as 1552 BCE, as documented in the *Ebers Papyrus*, an Ancient Egyptian compilation of medical texts, and Alexander the Great was said to have conquered the island of Socotra in the Indian Ocean purely to get hold of aloe plants. By the 10th century CE, aloe was found in Europe, and a hundred years later it was mentioned in traditional Chinese medicine texts.

Tips for Growing
Yellowing, red or orange leaves on an aloe can signify it is in too much sun, so move it out of direct sunlight to more dappled or part-shade. A regular application of liquid fertilizer through the summer will help to keep it healthy. The baby plants that can appear around the base of the mother plant are called pups; sever these with a section of root and plant into their own pots to grow on or give away.

How to Use
Aloe juice is widely sold by herbal suppliers as a preparation for aiding the digestion – it is a powerful laxative for short-term constipation – but these formulations have modified the neat sap to make it less irritating to the intestines.

CONTINUED OVERLEAF

It is not advised to take the fresh sap internally, and also avoid the yellow juice from the base of the leaf, known as bitter aloes and restricted in some countries.

For burns and stings, aloe is instantly cooling and soothing, with antibacterial and anti-inflammatory qualities. Simply cut off a fresh leaf and squeeze the clear sap onto the affected area, or cut open lengthways and scrape it out, repeating twice daily.

FROZEN ALOE CUBES

To make an aloe salve, blend together the sap from two aloe leaves with the petals from 8 fresh marigold flower heads (see page 96) and 1 tsp of raw honey; 10–15 drops of lavender essential oil will give a further antiseptic benefit. Pour the mix into an ice-cube tray and freeze, transferring the cubes to an airtight container in the freezer once solid. Take out as needed to rub onto burns and sunburned skin. Use within three months.

ALOYSIA CITRODORA

Lemon verbena

Lemon verbena is used more as a culinary than medicinal herb today, but it is helpful in pepping up the flavour of less palatable herbal infusions. The leaves are rich in lemon-scented volatile oils which perfume the garden.

Cultivation
A tender deciduous shrub, lemon verbena should be planted in a sunny spot with well-drained soil, or in a pot. Protect from frost.

A History of Healing
The oil is used in aromatherapy to soothe and relax, and is said to bring relief to conditions that cause gut and other muscle spasms. Traditionally, it was taken internally to reduce fever, but modern research is focusing on the oil's protective effects on nerve cells – it may benefit sufferers of dementia and Alzheimer's disease.

Tips for Growing
To keep growth compact and manageable, prune branches back to half their length in autumn, picking off and drying the leaves to use over winter.

How to Use
Use the leaves fresh or dried in tisanes, either on their own or to bring a lemon flavour to otherwise bitter or grassy herbs and herb mixtures. The infused syrup can be used in baking.

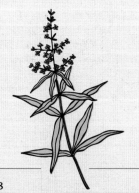

ORIGINS
South America

ALPINIA OFFICINARUM

Galangal *Gao Liang Jiang*

Although long used in Ayurvedic and traditional Chinese medicine preparations, galangal only arrived in Western Europe around a thousand years ago. It is similar in both appearance and effects to ginger (see page 246).

Caution
Large doses can cause irritation to the bowel.

Cultivation
Galangal requires humidity, a minimum temperature of 15°C (59°F), well-drained but rich soil and partial shade, but can also be grown as a house plant in a large pot. It will reach around 1m (3ft) in height in a pot, or 2m (6½ft) high when planted in the ground, with a spread of around 60cm–1.2m (2–4ft).

A History of Healing
All herbal traditions value galangal as a warming herb, to stimulate the digestion and relieve stomach pain, indigestion, flatulence and hiccups. Hildegard of Bingen thought it the 'spice of life', sent from God to prevent ill health.

Galangal has anti-inflammatory, antibacterial and antifungal properties and has been shown to be effective in the treatment of colds and yeast infections.

Harvesting
Lift the rhizomes (roots) of four- to six-year-old plants in autumn and use them fresh, or dry them to store.

How to Use
Prepare the rhizomes (roots) as a decoction or tincture and take to support the digestion or relieve nausea.

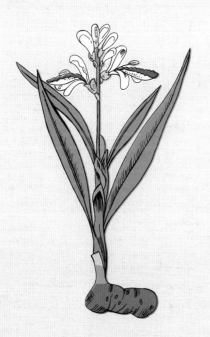

ALTHAEA OFFICINALIS

Marsh mallow *Mallow*

The marsh mallow is the superior species when the root of mallows are called for, but the leaves of other mallow species, such as common mallow (*Malva sylvestris*) and hollyhocks (*Alcea rosea*) can be used interchangeably with *Althaea*. The gloopy mucus found in marsh mallow roots is the original source of the squidgy confectionery that bears its name; boiled and whisked, it resembles whipped egg whites and can be used as a vegan alternative for them, for example, in meringues.

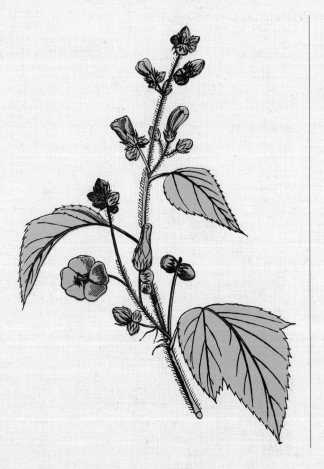

Caution
When taken internally, the demulcent effect will prevent the absorption of medicines and food for two hours after consuming the mallow, so time it appropriately.

Cultivation
As its name suggests, marsh mallow prefers moist soils, yet likes its aerial parts in the sunshine. In a border, simply water it frequently. A hardy herbaceous perennial, it can reach 1–2m (3–6½ft) tall and 1m (3ft) wide. Cut back old stems and mulch in late winter.

A History of Healing

Mallows are cited in almost every classical and medieval herbal, with uses for the leaves and roots ranging from eye ointments to easing childbirth, and from voiding poison to alleviating diarrhoea, dating back to the 3rd century BCE. Externally, poultices of the leaves were used to reduce inflammation. A simple, practical garden use of mallow suggested by Culpeper is as a soothing treatment for bee and wasp stings: the leaf is crushed and rubbed directly onto the sting site and will 'presently take away the pain, redness, and swelling that rise thereupon'.

Elizabeth Blackwell wrote that mallow was 'mollifying, digesting and soupling' – 'soupling' meaning that it was easy to take due to its slippery nature. Certainly marsh mallow's demulcent properties make it especially soothing for sore throats, coughs and an irritated bowel, and the dried roots were traditionally infused in sweet wine or powdered and made into lozenges to calm and coat inflamed mucous membranes of either or both. The peeled, fresh root is a time-honoured teething stick for babies.

Foraging

Mallows can often be found growing wild, especially in coastal areas. These are more likely to be *Malva* species or hollyhocks (*Alcea*) than *Althaea*, but as foraging laws permit only the use of the leaves, this does not matter. Avoid any with orange pustules on the leaves – this is a form of fungal plant disease called rust.

Harvesting

Pick leaves in summer just before the flowers form – the buds will be visible in the leaf axils – to use fresh or dry to store. Dig up a portion of the root in early autumn to use fresh or dry to store. Both are more mucilaginous when fresh but can be used dried.

How to Use

Crush and apply the leaves direct to the skin, or prepare as a poultice, to soothe any irritation, sting or rash. Hot- or cold-water infusions of the leaves serve as a soothing compress for sunburn, and can be drunk to coat a sore throat and ease a cough. They will also benefit gastric ulcers and other digestive upsets in small doses (larger quantities are laxative).

HONEYED MALLOW ROOTS

To soothe sore throats and tickly coughs, scrub and finely slice a small quantity of marsh mallow root and place in a small saucepan. Cover with honey (2–3 tbsp) and bring to the boil (the honey will froth up, so allow for this with the depth of the pan). Remove from the heat and leave to cool in the pan before eating. Consume within a day, as the roots will not store well.

AMMI VISNAGA

Khella *Visnaga, ammi, toothpick weed*

A herb more of interest for its isolated compounds than synergistic effect, *Ammi visnaga* is the source of khellin, a powerful antispasmodic from which the asthma drug Intal is derived.

Caution
Long-term use produces various side-effects, and the herb is restricted in some countries.

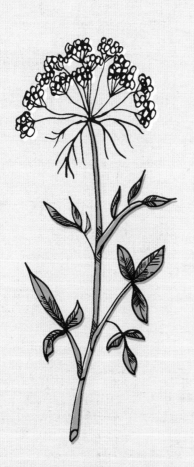

Cultivation
Khella is an annual or biennial grown from seed sown in spring. As it is only half-hardy, it needs well-drained soil in full sun and protection from frost. Plants will reach around 75–100cm (2½–3ft) tall and 45cm (18in) wide.

A History of Healing
Traditionally, khella has been used to alleviate the pain caused by kidney stones, and modern research has shown why it is effective in this respect: it relaxes the ureter so the trapped stone causes less pain to the surrounding area and also allows the stone to pass more easily into the bladder.

The dried flower stalks are sold as toothpicks in North Africa and Spain, and in Andalusia the herb was so valued that it came third only to gold and silver in the saying, *'Oro, plata, visnaga o nada!'* ('Gold, silver, visnaga or nothing!').

Other Uses
Ammi visnaga is from the same family as the popular annual bishop's weed (*Ammi majus*), and both make attractive cut flowers. *A. majus* is less medicinally helpful, but is used externally in preparations for psoriasis.

How to Use
Consult a qualified herbalist before taking khellin for either kidney stones or to reduce the incidence of asthma attacks.

ANETHUM GRAVEOLENS
(SYN. *PEUCEDANUM GRAVEOLENS*)

Dill

Dill is more widely known as a culinary herb, especially for its use in pickles and gravlax, but can be an effective digestive aid as well. It also makes a pretty cut flower.

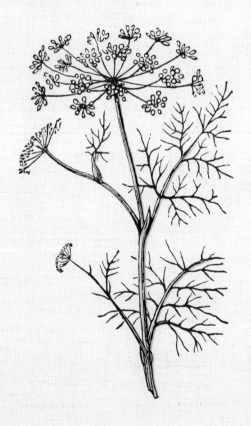

Cultivation
Widely naturalized in the Mediterranean region, this slender annual grows up to 1m (3ft) tall and is frost hardy. Sow seed in spring, making successional sowings for a regular supply of leaves.

A History of Healing
Dill is one of the gentlest herbal reliefs of stomach griping and pains, so gentle in fact that it is an ingredient of gripe water given to babies. It has long been used to treat flatulence and the pain that trapped wind can cause. Culpeper wrote, 'it is a gallant expeller of wind'. It is also a mild diuretic.

Its name derives from the Norse word *dylla*, which means 'to lull' or 'soothe'. In the Middle Ages, it was a commonly used herb against witchcraft, and burning dill was believed to clear thunderclouds.

Tips for Growing and Harvesting
Thin the seedlings to allow each plant plenty of space; they will flower and set seed prematurely if too crowded. Pick the leaves as needed, and harvest and dry the seeds.

How to Use
A hot- or cold-water infusion of the fresh leaves or seeds is a useful natural remedy for various symptoms of indigestion or cramping due to period pain, especially in combination with cramp bark (see page 243). The seeds, crushed slightly first, are more effective than the leaves. An infusion taken by nursing mothers can help a baby's digestion. Alternatively, incorporate the fresh leaves into the diet, adding them to salads and/or dishes with potatoes, fish or cream.

ANGELICA ARCHANGELICA

Angelica

Parkinson held angelica to be the most useful of all herbs, and in folklore it is the cure for all evils, associated with St Michael the Archangel. Angelica is an ingredient in gin, Benedictine and many other liqueurs and cordials often served as aperitifs or digestifs, pointing to its carminative effects.

Caution
Contraindicated during pregnancy. Contact or use can increase skin sensitivity to light and may cause phytophotodermatitis (irritation and/or inflammation caused when a plant's sap on the skin reacts with sunlight) or dermatitis.

Cultivation
Angelica prefers a moist, rich soil in full or partial shade. A biennial or short-lived perennial, it flowers in the second year of growth but will happily seed around the garden. An attractive sculptural plant for the back of the border, it reaches around 2m (6½ft) tall and 1m (3ft) wide.

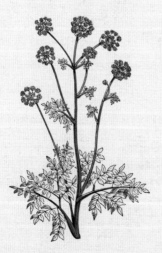

A History of Healing
As befits the 'angelic herb', angelica has traditionally been prescribed for bronchial complaints, fevers, digestive and menstrual problems, rheumatism and even 'the bitings of mad dogs', according to Gerard.

Bergapten, an isolated compound from the plant, has been shown effective in the treatment of psoriasis when combined with ultraviolet light therapy. Herbalists use angelica as an all-round tonic and also to stimulate the circulation in the treatment of Buerger's disease (narrowed arteries of the hands and feet).

Foraging
When foraging, be completely sure of making a correct identification, as angelica resembles various poisonous plants, such as hemlock (*Conium maculatum*) and giant hogweed (*Heracleum mantegazzianum*).

How to Use
Use the roots of the first year's growth, harvested in late autumn and dried before using, to prepare decoctions or infuse the seeds in hot water. Either preparation can be drunk to aid digestion.

The young stems can be candied or stewed with rhubarb, the leaves and flower buds eaten raw or cooked.

ANGELICA SINESIS (SYN. A. POLYMORPHA VAR. SINENSIS)

Dong quai *Dang Gui, Chinese angelica*

Dong quai comes second only to ginseng as a therapeutic herb in traditional Chinese medicine. Taken daily by many Chinese women, it is considered to have a stronger tonic effect than its European cousin *Angelica archangelica*.

Caution
Contraindicated during pregnancy and for heavy menstrual bleeding, bleeding disorders and diarrhoea. May interact negatively with blood-thinning medication.

Cultivation
A hardy perennial, dong quai prefers a moist, rich soil and dappled shade. It will reach around 1m (3ft) tall and 50cm (20in) wide. Cut back old stems in late winter.

A History of Healing
Chinese folk medicine uses dong quai primarily in cooking, including in a chicken soup traditionally given to women after childbirth. It is also taken as a tonic, stimulating the digestion and circulation and regulating menstrual flow.

Foraging
Dong quai resembles various poisonous plants, such as hemlock (*Conium maculatum*) and giant hogweed (*Heracleum mantegazzianum*), so be completely sure of its identification when foraging.

How to Use
The dried roots can be chopped and cooked and made into a soup, decoction or tincture.

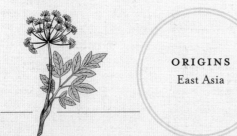

ORIGINS
East Asia

ANTHRISCUS CEREFOLIUM

Chervil *French parsley*

Chervil is a valuable culinary herb – one of the *fines herbes* of French cuisine – having a cleansing and diuretic effect on the body and imparting a fresh spring feeling after the sluggishness of winter. Culpeper recorded that 'it is good to help provoke urine', but it is little written of elsewhere, being considered a salad rather than a medicinal herb.

Cultivation
Rich yet light soil suits chervil best, in dappled or partial shade. An annual, it will grow to around 45cm (18in) tall and 25cm (10in) wide. Sow in late summer and protect with a cloche over winter as warm-weather sowings tend to run to seed early.

How to Use
The abundant leaves of chervil in early spring make it an ideal ingredient in any spring cleansing tonic/tea or early spring salad to aid the digestion. It doesn't dry well, making it a truly seasonal remedy. The fresh leaves can be infused in cold water or, better still, eaten raw. In cooking, add just before serving to best preserve the flavour.

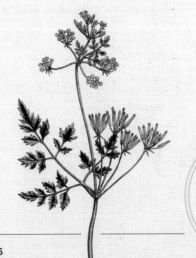

ORIGINS
Europe,
West Asia

ARCTIUM LAPPA

Burdock *Beggar's buttons, lappa, Niu Bang Zi*

Burdock will be well known to walkers for its hooked burrs, or seedheads – the species name *lappa* is from the Latin *lappare*, meaning 'to seize'. Culpeper noted that these also made for good rural weaponry: 'the little boys…pull off the burs to throw and stick upon each other', and in fact it was the tenacious hooks of burdock that inspired the invention of Velcro.

Caution
Burdock is a member of the Asteraceae family and should be avoided by anyone with allergies to these plants.

Cultivation
Burdock prefers moist soil in sun or dappled shade. It is a biennial, and is best planted in a wilder area of the garden where it can self-seed. It grows to around 1.5m (5ft) tall and 1m (3ft) wide.

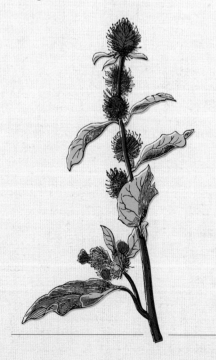

A History of Healing
Burdock is held to be powerfully detoxifying in both Western and Chinese herbal traditions. In Europe it was taken for gout, kidney stones and to break fevers. In both Western and Chinese traditions it was used to cleanse the body of toxins and therefore improve any chronic conditions affected by them, such as acne, abscesses, eczema and psoriasis.

Although all parts of the plant can be used, the root is considered to have the strongest effect. Burdock's young stems and root, which is known as *gobo* in Japan, feature in many Asian cuisines. Burdock is rarely taken in isolation, but combined with other herbs such as in the root beer and temperance drink dandelion and burdock.

Harvesting
Lift the roots in autumn when they can be eaten fresh as a vegetable or dried to use in remedies.

How to Use
A bitter herb, burdock is helpful to the digestion and will also cleanse the body of toxins. Combine with dandelion root (see page 226) in a decoction or cordial.

ARNICA MONTANA

Arnica *Leopard's bane*

Arnica is a small plant with sunny yellow daisy-like flowers that is increasingly under threat in its natural mountain habitats. The origin of its common name leopard's bane is unknown; the name is also sometimes applied to the toxic aconitum.

Caution
Arnica is a member of the Asteraceae family and should be avoided by anyone with allergies to these plants. For external use only; it may cause contact dermatitis. Restricted use in some countries.

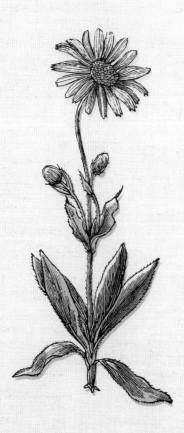

Cultivation
This hardy perennial alpine requires good air circulation and soil drainage, especially in winter. It can be grown in a rock garden or similar setting, reaching up to 60cm (2ft) when in flower, 10cm (4in) without flowers, and has a spread of just 15cm (6in).

A History of Healing
Arnica has long been used as a remedy for bruises and sprains and a gargle for mouth inflammations. Historically it was also taken as a tea (infusion) for heart problems, such as angina. It is thought that, when applied to an area of bruising, arnica increases blood flow and the rate of reabsorption of internal bleeding, thus accelerating the healing of the bruise.

Modern research has shown that arnica is extremely toxic when taken internally, and can cause contact dermatitis when applied externally. Homeopathic medicines of arnica are not toxic, as the dose of the active ingredient is so low, but consult a herbalist if in any doubt.

Harvesting
Pick the flowers when they are in full bloom, and dry before use.

How to Use
Dried flowers can be infused in oil, lotions and balms and applied to bruises but only on unbroken skin. Patch-test any preparations first.

ORIGINS
Europe, Asia

ARTEMISIA

Sweet wormwood, wormwood and mugwort

The *Artemisia* genus comprises around three hundred different species, many of them of interest for their medicinal or culinary properties. The wormwoods and mugworts have the longest herbal histories, which are detailed below, but the group also includes the culinary herb tarragon and some attractive ornamentals, with silvery, finely cut foliage and dainty flowers.

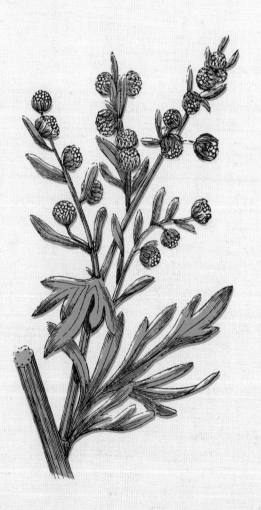

Caution
Some *Artemisia* species are toxic, addictive or carcinogenic in the short and/or long term. All are contraindicated during pregnancy and breastfeeding. Consult a qualified herbalist before taking any preparations involving *Artemisia* and be completely sure of any relevant plant identification. *Artemisia* is a member of the Asteraceae family and should be avoided by anyone with allergies to these plants.

Cultivation
Sweet wormwood (*A. annua*), wormwood (*A. absinthium*) and mugwort (*A. vulgaris*) are all hardy species, reaching around 1–1.5m (3–5ft) in height and half that in spread. They prefer well-drained soil in full sun.

A History of Healing
Sweet wormwood, also known as sweet Annie and Qing Hao, is an annual artemisia used in traditional Chinese medicine as a herb to break fevers and otherwise cool the body. However, in the 1970s and '80s, researchers isolated its key active constituent, artemisinin, and discovered its powerful antimalarial properties.

Artemisinin continues to play an important part in malaria prevention and treatments today.

Wormwood is perhaps the most notorious of the *Artemisia* genus because of its association with the alcoholic beverage absinthe. The species name *absinthium* means 'without sweetness', and this is a truly bitter herb, so it does have a beneficial effect on the digestion. Some research has indicated that it may have a use in treating inflammatory bowel disease. It is a principal aromatic in vermouth: the name vermouth derives from the German for wormwood, *Wermut*.

Absinthe, whose key ingredient is wormwood essential oil, was invented in the late 18th century and soon embraced by the creative community, especially in Paris. The Green Fairy, as it was called, was favoured by painters, musicians and writers, including Manet, Toulouse-Lautrec, Van Gogh, Picasso and Hemingway, perhaps for the inspiration it brought about through its hallucinogenic qualities. However, absinthe is also addictive and contains the highly toxic substance thujone, which, in excess, damages the central nervous system. Before this was even discovered there were public concerns about the violence that absinthe could cause – it was implicated in various crimes, including murder – and it was banned in Switzerland in 1908, with many other countries following suit. Wormwood is still an ingredient of vermouth, however, and is safe to drink in this respect.

Mugwort is the mildest in effect of the herbal artemisias and has a long history. Dioscorides associated it with the Greek goddess Artemis, and it was used for problems with menstruation and childbirth in Western, Chinese and Ayurvedic traditions, though some of the uses are contradictory between the traditions. As a bitter herb it can be used to stimulate the digestion; in TCM it is known as moxa for its use in moxibustion, a process by which herbs are rolled into a cigar shape (a smudge stick), lit at one end and pressed briefly to the skin on acupuncture points, to warm them.

Since the time of the Druids, mugwort has been used to banish evil spirits and it is said a pillow of mugwort will drive away nightmares and give the sleeper lucid dreams. It is an effective insect repellent when burned or hung in bunches around doorways or used in moth-repelling sachets. The Romans valued mugwort for soothing sore feet, and would plant it alongside roads so that the soldiers could pick sprigs to put in their sandals. The 17th-century herbalist William Coles even asserted that, 'If a footman take mugwort and put it in his shoes in the morning he may go forty miles by noon, and not be weary.'

How to Use

Flowering tops and leaves, fresh or dried, of mugwort can be added in a low dose to other bitter herbs in a tincture or occasionally prepared as a weak hot-water infusion to benefit the digestion.

ASTRAGALUS MEMBRANACEUS

Astragalus *Milk vetch, Huang Qi, Pak Kei*

A popular ingredient of soups, porridge (congee) and teas in Asia, astragalus is a key component of traditional Chinese medicine and used in many formulas, often in combination with dong quai (see page 85). It is an adaptogen and believed to help the body resist the cold.

Cultivation
Astralagus prefers a light, sandy, slightly alkaline soil in full sun. A fully hardy perennial, it reaches around 50cm (20in) in height and 40cm (16in) in spread.

A History of Healing
Astragalus has long been widely used in TCM as a tonic herb, one that warms the body and increases immunity and the body's ability to resist or adapt to external influences; it is as popular as ginseng (see page 178) in this regard. It is thought to benefit the circulation and increase energy, stamina and endurance and, perhaps because of the latter, is seen as a young or active person's herb. It is also used in cases of excessive sweating, such as night sweats, and is believed to encourage blood flow to the surface of the body, allowing it to cool down.

Recent research has shown that astragalus may have potential as a treatment for kidney disease, delaying the need for dialysis. It has also shown some benefit in promoting a faster recovery in cancer patients when taken concurrently with chemotherapy or radiotherapy.

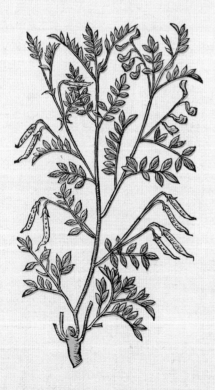

Harvesting
Lift the roots of four-year-old plants in autumn and dry before storing or using.

How to Use
The roots have a sweet taste that combines well with cinnamon – a decoction of the root with a quarter quantity of cinnamon makes a stimulating, warming drink. A decoction with dong quai is more strengthening. For night sweats, prepare a tincture of the roots. The roots can also be dry-fried (add a little honey, if liked, and serve with porridge).

BERBERIS VULGARIS

Barberry

Barberries are extremely sour but healthful berries that contain high levels of vitamin C. They can be dried (when they are known as *zereshk*), juiced and added to drinks, or preserved in a jam or jelly. The bark is also widely used in herbal medicine.

Caution
Contraindicated during pregnancy. All parts of the plant except the ripe berries are toxic if ingested directly. Berberis is a host of wheat rust and planting may be prohibited in some countries.

Cultivation
Barberry is a deciduous shrub with dense, thorny stems, growing to around 2m (6½ft) tall and 1.2m (4ft) wide. It is tolerant of most soils and situations. Prune in summer to keep it to size if necessary.

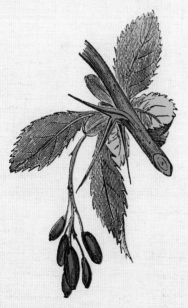

A History of Healing
Barberry is an interesting example of the application of the Doctrine of Signatures (see page 19), its yellow bark thought to indicate an effectiveness against liver complaints and jaundice. Culpeper held it an excellent purgative, and Ayurvedic treatments also use it as a cleansing herb, to rid the body of toxins and waste, often paired with turmeric (see page 118).

Berberine, an isolated alkaloid of barberry, has a strong antibacterial action that is used in Asia as a treatment for some eye diseases and also diarrhoea – indeed, the bark has an overall beneficial effect on the digestion as an antibacterial, anti-inflammatory, astringent and bitter herb that is also thought to strengthen the intestinal wall. Berberine has been shown to prevent bacteria from attaching themselves to the body's cell walls, enhancing its reputation as a cleansing herb.

Harvesting
The berries are ripe in autumn. Bark can be gathered in spring or autumn; the bark of the root is considered marginally more potent but the stem bark is also effective and easier to harvest.

How to Use
Dry the ripe berries and sprinkle them over salads or rice, or preserve them with other autumn berries and hips to make a hedgerow jelly. Prepare the bark in a decoction or tincture.

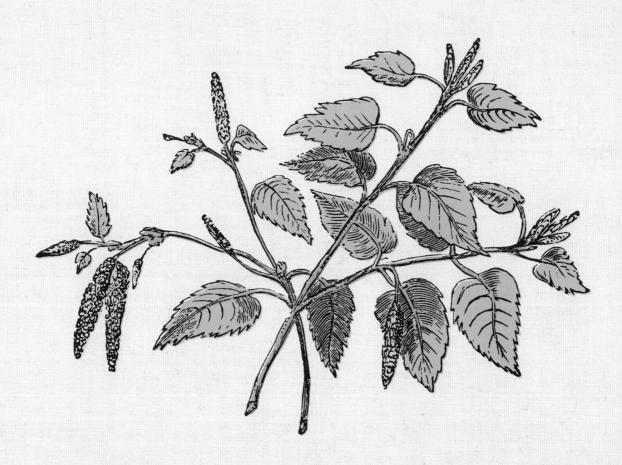

BETULA PENDULA (SYN. *B. VERRUCOSA*, *B. ALBA*)

Silver birch

Iconic in the wild and gardens for its white bark, the name birch is possibly derived from its Sanskrit name *bhurga*, which means 'tree on which the bark is used for writing'. Birch sap, also known as birch water, has been drunk for centuries in the northernmost reaches of Europe and is now gaining popularity as a health drink.

Cultivation

Birch is a pioneer species, a tree that grows fast and tall, colonizing most soils as a first step in a return to woodland, before dying relatively young to make way for beeches and oaks. Deciduous, it will reach 10–25m (33–82ft) tall and 4–10m (13–33ft) wide.

A History of Healing

Silver birch is a diuretic, traditionally used as a spring cleansing herb, purifying the blood and ridding the body of urinary infections and cystitis, as well as having a beneficial action on rheumatism, gout, chronic skin disorders, hair loss and dandruff. Birch tar oil, which is distilled from the leaves, is antiseptic and used externally on psoriasis and eczema. In Russia, silver birch is held to be a highly useful medicinal plant, especially in cases of arthritis, and modern research has focused on its potential in this regard and as a treatment for cancer.

How to Use

The leaves can be picked in spring and dried or prepared as a cleansing hot-water infusion or as an infused oil to massage into areas affected by cellulite. Drinking the sap has a similar cleansing effect.

TAPPING BIRCH SAP

Birch sap is harvested in spring, as the sap rises through the tree, preparing to put on its new leaves. A small hole is drilled into the bark and a pipe inserted. As the sap rises through the tree, some of it diverts down the pipe from where it can be collected in a bottle. The speed and force of this flow can be surprising, and it is best to be tutored in the correct technique by a foraging expert before attempting it, as a wrong step can fatally wound the tree.

BORAGO OFFICINALIS

Borage *Starflower*

Bees love the star-shaped, vivid blue flowers of borage – it is possible to buy borage honey – which make eye-catching additions to savoury dishes and drinks such as Pimm's.

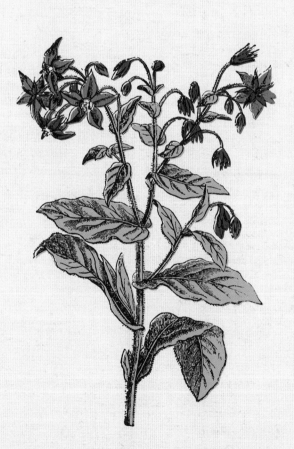

Caution
Borage leaves are known to contain alkaloids, which are toxic when consumed in quantity. Limit use to the flowers and proprietary seed oil, to avoid them completely, or eat only the young leaves occasionally in spring. Older leaves can be a skin irritant. Some countries restrict its use.

Cultivation
Grow borage once, and it will happily self-seed around the garden thereafter; Elizabeth Blackwell wrote that it 'grows frequently as a Weed in Gardens'. An annual, it can reach up to 1m (3ft) in height and 30cm (12in) in spread, less if growing in paving cracks and poorer soils. Sow seed directly outside in spring and protect young plants from slugs. Borage is a useful companion plant in the garden, attracting pollinators and deterring some pests.

A History of Healing
Borage seed oil is known to contain high levels of gamma-linolenic acid (GLA), and is rich in healthy polyunsaturated fats, which are known to promote healthy brain functioning and regulate hormones and inflammatory responses in the body. This may explain the plant's reputation

among herbal authors, from Pliny the Elder to Parkinson, as a herb to improve the mood and alleviate depression. Gerard wrote, 'the floures [flowers] in sallads' and other preparations could be used 'for the comfort of the heart, to drive away sorrow, & increase the joy of the minde.' Blackwell attributed the same qualities to the leaves, which she considered 'Esteemed cordial, comforting the Heart.'

Harvesting

Continual picking of the flowers will encourage more to be produced, but leave some for the bees. The leaves are covered in tiny hairs that can irritate the skin, so wear gloves. Use the flowers fresh, or dry until they feel papery and will not roll up between the fingers.

How to Use

Young leaves, before they turn hairy, can be steamed or wilted, as for other leafy greens such as nettle or spinach, but they should be eaten only occasionally. Infused in hot water with lemon balm, they make a tisane to aid digestion and drive away melancholy. Again, consume only occasionally.

Add the fresh flowers to salads, use them to decorate cakes, savoury dishes and drinks (remove the black stamens, if preferred) or make ice cubes with them. They have a cucumber-like taste that doesn't tend to complement sweet dishes. Scatter the dried flowers over rice dishes, porridge and muesli, or infuse them in cold water.

BOSWELLIA SERRATA

Boswellia *Indian frankincense, Indian olibanum, sallaki*

Related to true frankincense, boswellia is a deciduous tree which exudes a clear gold-coloured gum resin from its bark. This resin is collected and used fresh, or dried for storage.

A History of Healing

Boswellia's use as an anti-inflammatory and antiseptic treatment, especially for infections of the mouth and throat, dates back thousands of years. It is powerfully astringent and when used as a mouthwash or gargle, it can be helpful for mouth ulcers, gum disease and sore throats.

Recent research has focused on boswellia's anti-inflammatory properties, with initial results suggesting it may have potential as a treatment for arthritis, inflammatory bowel disease and asthma. It is also believed to have a stabilizing effect on blood sugar levels in people with Type 2 diabetes.

How to Use

Boswellia is not recommended as a home remedy, and should be taken only under the direction of a qualified herbalist.

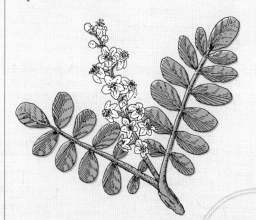

ORIGINS
India

CALENDULA OFFICINALIS

Marigold *Pot marigold, goldes*

There are many cultivars of marigolds, offering different colour and petal variations, but *Calendula officinalis* is the best to grow for both herbal use and for the benefit of bees and other beneficial insects they attract. Other plants with the common name marigold include *Tagetes*, which should not be used in place of *Calendula*.

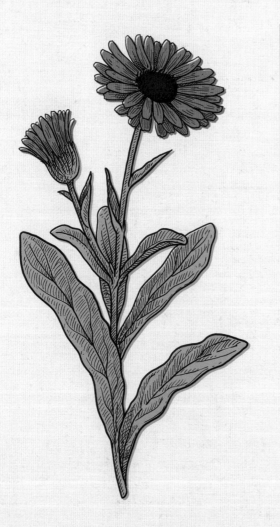

Caution
Marigold is a member of the Asteraceae family and should be avoided by anyone with allergies to these plants.

Cultivation
Marigolds are happy little plants, technically short-lived perennials but most often grown as annuals, though they will flower well into autumn and winter given some protection from the cold. Sow seeds in spring, pinching out the seedling tip to encourage bushy growth. They can reach 40–50cm (16–20in) in height and spread and prefer well-drained soil in full sun.

A History of Healing
Predominantly used in the Western herbal tradition, marigold is the primary plant for healing all manner of skin conditions. It is antiseptic, antibacterial and astringent, making it an effective external remedy for cuts, grazes

and varicose veins, especially when combined with witch hazel (see page 142). It is also calming, soothing and softening for sunburn, dry skin, nappy rash and cradle cap. Research has shown it to be effective in healing skin ulcers and dermatitis, and it is now of scientific interest for its potential in alleviating skin cancers.

Marigold is also mildly bitter and therefore helpful for the digestion when taken internally, and soothing to inflammatory gastric conditions such as ulcers, diverticulitis and colitis. It is considered detoxifying, cleansing the liver and gallbladder and helping to rid the body of waste toxins that can be the underlying cause of chronic skin complaints and cellulite.

The petals are edible, if not particularly flavourful, and brighten up salads and rice dishes, as well as imparting a yellow/orange colour to risottos, cheeses and cream dishes. Culpeper wrote that they were 'much used in possets, broths and drink, as a comforter of the heart and spirits' which could be either from their tonic effect or simply because of the sunny colour imbued from the petals. As a flower used in ancient religious ceremonies, it gained the name Mary's gold, for the Virgin Mary, from which the name marigold has been corrupted.

Harvesting

Pick the flowers regularly, on a dry day, to encourage continual production through the summer, and dead-head any flowers that were missed. Lay out the complete flower heads in the sun for an hour or so before moving to a warm, dry but not so sunny spot to dry them completely without them losing their colour. They can be stored either as whole flower heads or the petals can be picked off.

How to Use

Mix dried flower heads with other herbs and use in tisanes, or sprinkle fresh or dried petals over food. The dried petals can also be infused into oil to use externally on skin complaints, or mixed with aloe vera gel in a soothing frozen salve (see page 78). A tincture of the petals can also be taken in the case of chronic skin conditions.

Marigold oil or salve is sufficiently gentle to use on a baby's skin for rashes and dry skin when in the correct formulation – use a proprietary marigold preparation or see page 63.

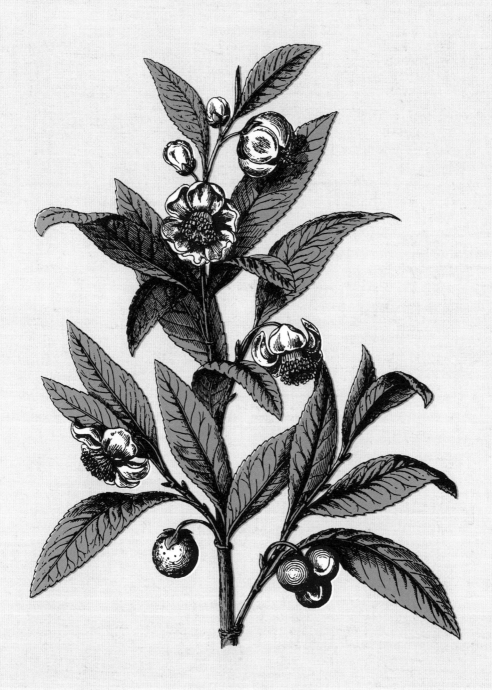

ORIGINS
China

CAMELLIA SINENSIS (SYN. THEA SINENSIS)

Tea

Green tea is the steamed and dried leaves of this plant. It has more health benefits than black tea, which is most commonly drunk in the West, and is made by fermenting and drying the leaves.

Cultivation

The world's biggest tea-growing countries are China, India and Kenya, but there is a successful tea plantation in Cornwall, UK. Tea prefers rich, moist soil in sun or partial shade and, while it is frost hardy, it will not withstand long periods of cold, wet weather. A tea plant can reach 6m (20ft) tall and 4m (13ft) wide, but regular picking can keep it to 1m (3ft) tall and 60cm (2ft) wide.

A History of Healing

Tea is used in both traditional Chinese medicine and Ayurvedic herbalism to treat cardiovascular and coronary problems. It is thought that green tea helps to lower blood pressure and cholesterol levels and prevent arteriosclerosis. A cooled, weak infusion of tea has also long been used to bathe the eyes, and in the absence of anything better to use, tea's astringency makes it suitable for first-aid treatment of burns.

It is known that tea leaves contain compounds called catechins that are anti-inflammatory, and current research is focusing on their ability to regulate blood glucose levels, especially in the case of Type 2 diabetes. Tea may also have a positive effect on the mind and memory, delaying the onset of symptoms in conditions such as Parkinson's or Alzheimer's diseases, but further research is needed.

Harvesting

Leaves can be harvested once the plant is three years old. It is believed in China that the leaves harvested in spring contain the most health benefits, but they can be picked throughout the year and then dried before use.

How to Use

Prepare dried green leaves as tea, either on their own or in combination with other herbs. Take inspiration from the tea ceremonies of China and Japan, and use the opportunity to have a mindful break while brewing and drinking the tea.

CAPSICUM ANNUUM

Chilli pepper *Bell pepper, sweet pepper, chilli*

Chillies can be a divisive food, with some people loving their heat and others detesting it, but with the huge variety of chilli peppers available, from the hot to the very mild, everyone can benefit from their therapeutic qualities.

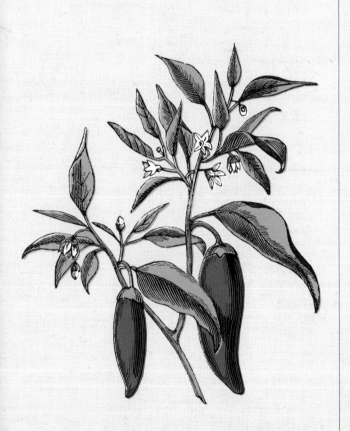

Cultivation

Chillies need plenty of sun and heat over a long growing season for them to do well, but they can be grown on windowsills, sunny patios or in greenhouses or polytunnels in temperate climates. Look for varieties specifically bred for a cooler climate if growing outdoors. Chillies should be sown in mid-winter in a heated propagator, or buy young plants. Plants grown under cover benefit from regular misting, to aid pollination. Specialist chilli farms will have the widest selection of varieties.

A History of Healing

Mayan and Aztec healing traditions have used peppers for thousands of years to treat diarrhoea and other bacterial infections, especially of the gut. The leaves were chewed for toothache. Chillies are also used to preserve food. First brought to Europe in the 15th century, their heat took many by surprise – until then black pepper (see page 186) and ginger (see page 246) had been the spiciest foods available. Parkinson writes in his *Theatrum Botanicum* that chillies 'are hot and dry in the fourth degree, and beyond it if there be any beyond it, and are so fiery hot and sharpe biting in tast, that they burne and enflame the mouth and throate so extreamely that it is hardly to be endured.'

Despite this, chillies soon found favour both in the kitchen and the apothecary's cabinet, and were used for treating digestive disorders and neutralizing the effects of other foods: Elizabeth Blackwell wrote that chilli was 'much used as a Sauce for any Thing that is flatulent and Windy'. The spice was also used to treat cold and colds, warming the body and stimulating poor circulation.

Capsaicin, which is the main therapeutic compound in chillies and gives them their heat, is used in its extracted form in preparations to treat osteoarthritis.

Harvesting
A green chilli is mature and ready to harvest when it feels firm to a gentle squeeze around the base of the stalk, and ripe (and thus sweeter and fruitier) when it changes colour. Pick at either stage to eat fresh, but in order to dry chillies, wait until they ripen. Chillies can be threaded onto a string by piercing the base of the stalk with a needle, then hung up in a warm, sunny spot until completely dried.

How to Use
The easiest option is to use chillies in food dishes, either in fresh or dried form (flakes or powdered). The more frequently chilli is consumed, the higher one's heat tolerance gets. Adding chilli to infusions or hot chocolate – the milk will help to neutralize some of the heat, allowing for a bigger dose of chilli without the fire – will also stimulate the circulation and digestion.

For cold and flu symptoms, chilli added to teas or broths can alleviate congestion, or for a sore throat, gargle diluted lemon juice with a pinch of chilli powder (add honey, if liked). Massage an infused oil with chilli into aching joints and muscles as both a mild pain relief and to stimulate the circulation to the area, helping to clear inflammation (see page 48).

CHILLI VARIETIES
The species includes all peppers from the not-at-all-spicy bell peppers to the almost dangerously hot chillies. The heat of a chilli is measured using the Scoville scale, with more Scoville Heat Units (SHU) indicating a hotter chilli. Plant breeders competing to cultivate the hottest chilli in the world tend to use the Scotch Bonnet or habanero types; the habanero 'Carolina Reaper' measures at over 2 million SHU.

Habanero chillies are the best for drying, flaking or powdering, as their flesh is thin and they have plenty of heat. For a more substantial, vegetable-type chilli, there are plenty of options that also offer a more complex flavour profile, such as the notably fruity and smoky 'Poblano' (c.700 SHU), the crunchy 'Apple Crisp' (c.400 SHU), which can be eaten raw like an apple, or 'Hungarian Hot Wax' (6,000 SHU).

CARUM CARVI

Caraway

Probably the spice with the longest cultivation history in Europe, caraway is a common flavouring for cheese, bread and cabbage dishes in German, Austrian and Jewish cookery. It only really features in the UK in the form of seedcake, which the British cookery writer Elizabeth David suggested was vastly improved by the addition of ground almonds, to make it less dry.

Cultivation
Rich, well-drained soil in sun or partial shade suits this biennial (it flowers and sets seed in its second year). A hardy plant, caraway will grow to up to 1m (3ft) tall and 30cm (12in) wide.

A History of Healing
Caraway seeds contain carminative and antispasmodic qualities which, according to Culpeper, made them 'a most admirable remedy, for those that are troubled with wind' for thousands of years. In medieval Europe they were especially popular in the form of comfit sweets, sugar-coated seeds nibbled after meals to ease indigestion and sweeten the breath. Mild enough for children and babies, caraway infusions were used to treat colic and griping. Seedcakes were traditionally baked to mark the end of the sowing of the wheat in spring.

Culpeper suggested the root was 'better food than the parsnip; it is pleasant and comfortable to the stomach, and helps digestion.' Caraway's clean, aniseed taste is also used to flavour toothpaste and mouthwashes.

Tips for Growing
Caraway plants have a long taproot, so will grow best in light soil or in a pot with a depth of at least 30cm (12in).

How to Use
The seeds can be infused for a tisane; they also pair well with fennel seeds for an after-dinner hot drink. Sprinkle the seeds over food, especially as a topping to a loaf of home-made bread, or bake a seedcake. Add leaves to salads, and cook the root as a vegetable.

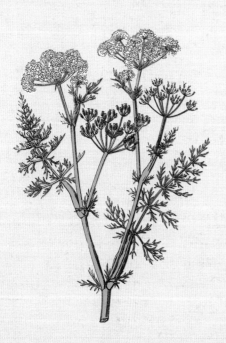

CENTAUREA CYANUS

Cornflower *Bachelor's buttons, casse-lunette (break glasses)*

Cornflowers make pretty cut flowers, as well as supplying petals for salads and cakes.

Caution
Cornflower is a member of the Asteraceae family and should be avoided by anyone with allergies to these plants.

Cultivation
Sow seeds in spring in a well-drained soil in sun. Plants will reach around 75cm (2½ft) in height and 20cm (8in) in spread. Picking the flowers regularly will encourage further production.

A History of Healing
Cornflowers were first recommended medicinally by Hildegard of Bingen, who advised taking an infusion in wine and applying a poultice for broken bones. Later, herbalists, following the Doctrine of Signatures (see page 19), used it as an ocular remedy – the bright blue flowers were thought to resemble healthy eyes. An infusion of cornflowers (*eau de casse-lunettes*) is still used in France today to treat eye complaints.

How to Use
A strained cold-water infusion can be used as an eyewash for conditions such as conjunctivitis. The petals are a bitter herb benefiting the digestion, and can be added fresh to savoury dishes.

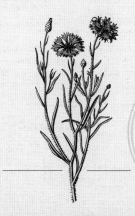

ORIGINS
Europe,
Mediterranean

CETRARIA ISLANDICA

Iceland moss

Iceland moss is actually a lichen, and because it grows in inhospitable climates where other plants are scarce, it is valuable as fodder for creatures such as reindeer and moose. Iceland moss is not the only moss or lichen to have a medicinal use; in the First World War, sphagnum moss was used in place of bandages when supplies ran low.

A History of Healing
The Northern European herbal tradition has valued Iceland moss since ancient times as a remedy for coughs, sore throats and other bronchial infections. Although it cannot be cultivated, it can be gathered all year round. Today it is known to be both a bitter herb and demulcent, which makes it almost unique among medicinal herbs, and therefore it is of potential help in relieving digestive conditions such as irritable bowel syndrome.

Foraging
Plants can be gathered whole, all year round, but they can be extremely scarce, so forage with consideration.

How to Use
Dry before preparing as a decoction or tincture.

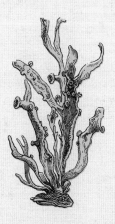

ORIGINS
Europe,
Arctic regions,
Australasia

CHAMAEMELUM NOBILE (SYN. *ANTHEMIS NOBILIS*)

Chamomile *Roman chamomile*

Chamomile was traditionally so widely grown in domestic gardens that Culpeper wrote that 'it is but lost time and labour to describe it'. It is a stalwart of the cottage garden as well as the herb garden, with its pretty daisy-like flowers and apple scent, used for fragrant seats, lawns and pathways where, as an old rhyme suggests, 'The more it is trodden, The more it will spread'.

German chamomile (*Matricaria chamomilla*) is a taller, bushier plant than the low-growing *Chamaemelum*. Either can be used for herbal remedies – the constituents and fragrance vary slightly but the effects are largely the same.

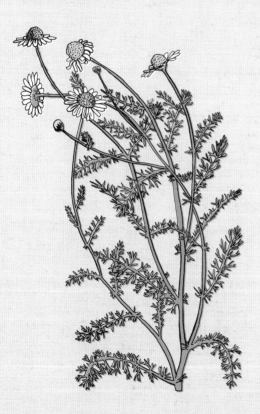

Caution
The essential oil should not be used during pregnancy. Chamomile is a member of the Asteraceae family and should be avoided by anyone with allergies to these plants.

Cultivation
A mat-forming, hardy perennial reaching 15–20cm (6–8in) high and 45cm (18in) wide, chamomile prefers light, well-drained soil in full sun. Cut back straggly stems while harvesting the flowers. The cultivar 'Treneague', sold for creating chamomile lawns, will not flower.

CHAMOMILE COCKTAILS
Prepare a chamomile sugar syrup using fresh or dried flowers; if you prefer, substitute honey for the sugar. To make a refreshing summer drink, mix 3 tbsp of chamomile syrup with around the same volume of sparkling wine or gin, and top up with tonic and a squeeze of lime. Serve over ice; use borage flower ice cubes (see page 95) if liked.

'Camomil [is used] in bathing to comfort and
strengthen the sound and to ease pains in the diseased.'

John Parkinson

A History of Healing

Chamomile has been used as a strewing herb for
thousands of years – its name derives from the
Greek for ground apple, referring to the scent
of the foliage. Its taste is somewhat different and
considerably more bitter than the fragrance,
but taken internally or externally it has been
applied to almost every medical complaint over
the centuries, with archaeological evidence
dating back to Neanderthal communities. Most
particularly, chamomile relaxes the mind and
soothes the digestion and skin.

Chamomile tea or baths have a sedative
effect, described by Mrs Grieve in her herbal
as 'wonderfully soothing' and the 'sole certain
remedy for nightmare', and the herb can ease
anxiety, stress and insomnia, calming the mind
when drunk before bedtime or at any time of
day. Roman chamomile is more bitter than the
German species, and thus more effective for
digestive complaints. Antispasmodic, it can
relieve griping, and it is also considered effective
for nausea, for 'summer diarrhoea in children'
according to Grieve, and indigestion – most
famously as suffered by Peter Rabbit. Anti-
inflammatory compounds in the flowers and
essential oil, which is a rather surprising vivid
blue colour, mean chamomile can help to relieve
itchy, dry and irritated skin, such as nappy rash
or sunburn.

Chamomile is also reputed to aid ailing
plants – it is said that putting chamomile near
sick plants will revive them, and that watering
seedlings with a chamomile infusion will
prevent damping off. Cut flowers certainly last
better in a vase of chamomile tea than in one
of plain water.

A CHAMOMILE BATH

Try harnessing the plant's relaxing properties
in a long soak. Add fresh or dried flowers
or an infusion of chamomile to bath water,
or use this two-in-one exfoliating scrub and
bath milk, which is especially beneficial to
dry and itchy skin conditions.

Mix 10 tbsp of rolled oats with 1 tsp of dried
chamomile flowers in a bowl, adding 10 drops
of lavender essential oil, if liked. Tip into the
middle of a muslin square and tie up into a
tight bundle. Soak the bag in the bath water
for a short while before using it to gently
cleanse the skin, returning the bag to the
water for the rest of bath time.

Harvesting

Pick the flowers once fully opened and dry in a
cool room out of direct sunlight.

How to Use

Fresh or dried flowers can be prepared as a hot-
water infusion, or infused into oil with lavender
for a moisturizing and soothing massage oil.
A relaxing bedtime tisane might include chamomile,
linden (see page 228) and lemon balm (see page
166). Relatively mild, chamomile flowers can
also be given to children as an infusion in water,
milk or honey, to calm frayed tempers and aid
sleep. A chilled facecloth soaked in a water
infusion was traditionally given to teething babies
to chew upon. Chamomile's volatile oils are very
easily lost in the steam rising from infusions, so
be sure to cover the cup or use a teapot.

CICHORIUM INTYBUS

Chicory *Succory*

Chicory is closely related to several other well-known species, including the salad vegetables radicchio, endive and Witloof chicory, and it is also an attractive plant for the back of the border.

Caution
Chicory is a member of the Asteraceae family and should be avoided by anyone with allergies to these plants. Chicory can lower blood sugar levels, so exercise caution if suffering from diabetes.

Cultivation
This fully hardy perennial reaches 1.5m (5ft), with a spread of around 50cm (20in). It prefers well-drained soil in full sun.

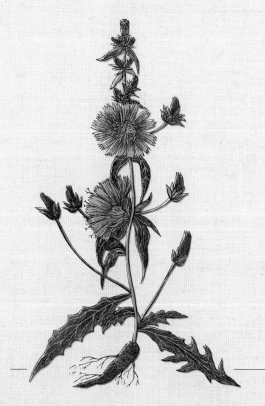

A History of Healing
Chicory is considered a cooling herb as well as a bitter herb for the digestion. Used in Ancient Egypt, China and India, it was probably one of the bitter herbs mentioned in the Bible (see page 57) and it still plays a part in the Passover meal today. Pliny the Elder recommended mixing the juice of chicory with rose oil and vinegar, for headaches. Galen used a sugar syrup of chicory, oats and rhubarb against liver complaints in his patients, probably recognizing, as John Evelyn did in his book *Acetaria* (1699), that chicory's bitterness makes it more 'grateful [pleasing] to the Stomach than the Palate'.

It is now known that the root comprises around 50 per cent inulin, a prebiotic substance that is highly beneficial for gut flora biodiversity.

Harvesting
Dig up the roots in spring or autumn: one-year-old growth has a slight caramel flavour and can be eaten as a vegetable. For use in remedies, harvest two-year-old roots.

How to Use
Add fresh leaves to salads or fry them in olive oil and garlic as an appetizer. The edible flowers can also be used to garnish savoury dishes. Prepare dried roots as a decoction or tincture, either in isolation or in combination with other bitter herbs, to benefit the digestion.

CINCHONA OFFICINALIS

Quinine *Peruvian bark*

Several species of the *Cinchona* genus have medicinal uses, but *C. officinalis* is the tree from which quinine is mostly extracted. Aside from its connection with Chelsea Physic Garden, quinine is also significant for being the first remedy that Samuel Hahnemann, the founder of the homeopathy discipline, tested on himself, leading to his formulation of the Law of Simples: 'Like cures like'.

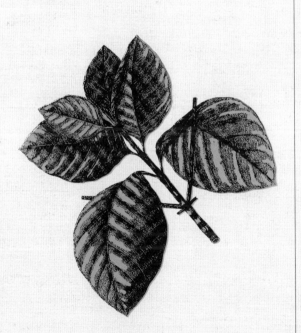

A History of Healing

The bark of this tropical species has been used for centuries by the indigenous people of South America for fevers and other infections, but it was not until European settlers discovered its efficacy as an antimalarial that *Cinchona* plantations were established. Quinine is one of the alkaloids that can be extracted from *Cinchona* bark, and it continued to be the primary malaria treatment until the First World War, when synthetic medicines began to replace it. However, as resistant strains of malaria develop, scientists are returning to quinine to treat the disease. The other main alkaloid it supplies is quinidine, a known cardiac depressant, which slows and regulates the heartbeat.

How to Use

Cinchona should only be taken under the supervision of a professional herbalist.

CINNAMOMUM

Cinnamon *Dalcini, Rou Gui*

The cinnamon genus includes three important species. *Cinnamomum zeylanicum*, also known as *C. verum*, is true cinnamon, although *C. cassia* (cassia) is often used as the culinary spice. *C. camphora* leaves produce camphor, the strongly bitter and aromatic herb that can be used in steam inhalations for decongestion and in skin liniments for joint or muscle pain. It is also found in lip salves for chapped lips, but should not be taken internally without advice from a qualified herbalist.

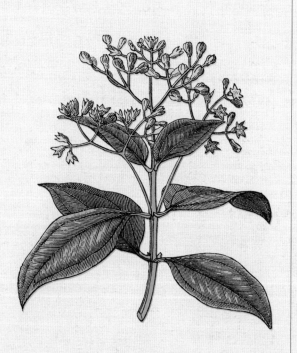

Cultivation

Cinnamon forms a large tree in its native tropical forests, but is coppiced to provide the best harvests, with the shoots being cut every other year. The outer bark is stripped away to reveal the inner bark, which is then peeled and dried into the characteristic quills. True cinnamon is fermented for 24 hours after cutting, whereas cassia is not. The leaves and bark can both be distilled, with the former making a delicate scented oil that is used in perfumery.

A History of Healing

Cinnamon is one of the most ancient recorded herbs, first appearing in traditional Chinese medicine documents in 2700 BCE and in Ancient Egypt in 1600 BCE. It is also mentioned in the Torah and is traditionally one of the spices in Jewish holy incense. As European countries expanded their colonies, access to suitable land in which to grow cinnamon was one of the primary concerns, and it was to gain control of the cinnamon trade that Portugal invaded Ceylon (now Sri Lanka) in the 16th century, although they ultimately ceded the monopoly to the Dutch East India Company by the 18th century.

All herbal traditions – TCM, Ayurveda and Western – use cinnamon as a warming herb to help treat cold and colds (often combined with ginger, see page 246) and to support the digestion. It is widely applied in herbal traditions for convalescence and is thought to stimulate the circulation. Most recently it has been discovered that cinnamon has a regulatory effect on blood sugar levels and it may therefore have potential as a treatment for Type 2 diabetes.

Buying Cinnamon

Most cinnamon sold in the spice section of supermarkets is cassia bark, and will be labelled as such. Cinnamon packets that do not declare the species origin are also likely to be cassia. *C. zeylanicum* is usually labelled as 'True' or 'Ceylon' cinnamon, but check with the manufacturer if in doubt; it is easily found from herbal suppliers and online.

How to Use

For the best therapeutic effect, use *C. zeylanicum*. Consult a qualified herbalist before taking significant quantities of cinnamon.

Cinnamon is a wonderfully warming herb, and is comforting during periods of cold and flu, or simply to warm up on a chilly day. Infuse it with other herbs in hot water, a hot chocolate or mulled juices/wine, where it can also temper the spiciness of chilli and ginger. For nausea or uncomfortable griping and diarrhoea, try a hot-water infusion of cinnamon with lemon juice and honey. A tincture is said to help relieve flatulence.

Cinnamon is a versatile spice that can be easily incorporated into the diet, sprinkled over porridge, used in baking or added to dhals and curries.

CITRUS

Lemon and bitter orange

Lemon (*Citrus* x *limon*) and bitter orange (*C.* x *aurantium*) are the more significant citrus species for herbal healing, but most citrus have some herbal application as well as being used in cooking and perfumery.

Cultivation
Citrus were introduced from Asia to the Mediterranean region around 1000 CE, and are now synonymous with that region and its climate. They need protection from prolonged cold and wet weather. Branches can be pruned back at any time of year to keep the plant's shape – they will naturally grow to a small or large tree, depending on the species.

A History of Healing
Citrus has traditionally been used more as a preventative medicine than a cure: as a nutritious, vitamin-rich fruit, it can support the immune system and help maintain a general level of good health. The age-old remedy of hot water with lemon and honey is still one of the best herbal preparations for sore throats and colds. Lemon's acidity is a useful antiseptic when used externally. Internally it has an antioxidant effect and is thought to strengthen the blood vessels.

The bitterness of the bitter orange has a beneficial effect on the digestion. Traditional Chinese medicine uses the unripe fruit, known as Zhi Shi, to regulate the digestion and alleviate bloating and flatulence. All bitter orange essential oils are thought to have a sedative effect, especially neroli, which is widely used to promote sleep and calm palpitations.

Harvesting
Most citrus fruit is harvested in winter, when the vitamin C levels are at their highest.

How to Use
A hot-water infusion of a slice of lemon with honey – with garlic (see page 74) and cinnamon (see page 108) for added benefit – is a warming, soothing drink to treat colds and flu, or at any time. Lemon essential oil can be dabbed onto mouth ulcers.

Bitter orange can be eaten (the Seville orange is widely believed to make the best marmalade), or infused in cold drinks for a bitter aperitif. The neroli essential oil, diluted and used for aromatherapy massage, can help to relieve tension and encourage relaxation.

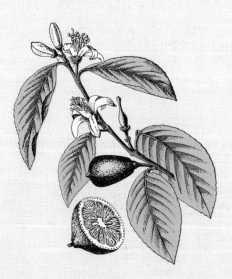

COMMIPHORA MYRRHA (SYN. C. MOLMOL)

Myrrh *Bola*

Familiar to many from the Christian nativity story, myrrh has been used since ancient times.

Caution
Contraindicated in pregnancy.

Cultivation
Myrrh forms a spiny shrub up to 5m (16½ft) tall and 1.5m (5ft) wide, but can be grown as an ornamental bonsai tree. It needs a minimum temperature of 10–15°C (50–59°F), so is best grown in a greenhouse or conservatory.

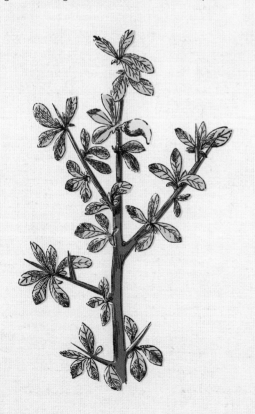

A History of Healing
Myrrh is one of the herbs used by the Ancient Egyptians for embalming, but it was also given to patients as a means of prolonging life and improving the skin tone. Myrrh is considered an aphrodisiac and a stimulant to intelligence in Ayurvedic medicine, as well as a general cleansing tonic. traditional Chinese medicine uses the resin, Mo Yao, as a herbal treatment for arthritis.

Myrrh is a flavouring in some toothpastes and also helps oral health due to its anti-inflammatory properties. It has antibacterial properties, too, and in Germany it is used to treat pressure sores caused by prosthetic limbs, providing a low level of pain relief.

Guggul (*Commiphora mukul*, syn. *C. wightii*) is a relative of myrrh that is widely revered in Ayurvedic healing as a herb to help in old age, remedying diseases associated with aging, and is used to rejuvenate the patient.

Harvesting
The branches, when cut, exude a resin, which is collected and left to dry into golden-coloured nuggets.

How to Use
Dab a tincture of myrrh directly onto mouth ulcers or dilute it as a mouth gargle (do not swallow). The diluted essential oil can be used for massage, especially around the sinuses to help alleviate congestion.

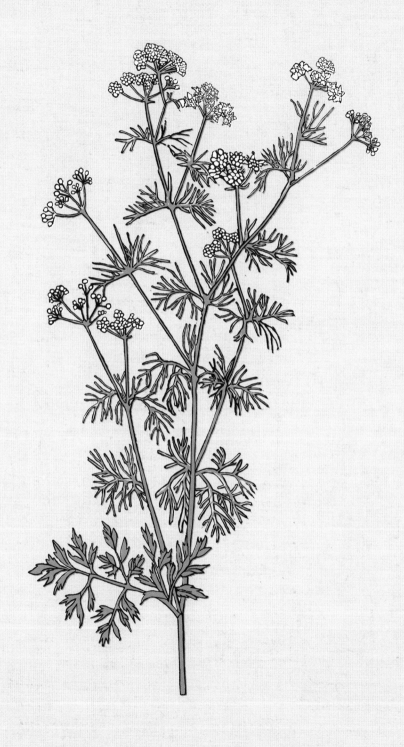

ORIGINS
South Europe,
North Africa,
Southwest Asia

CORIANDRUM SATIVUM

Coriander *Cilantro*

The leaves (often called cilantro) and seeds can be used interchangeably for herbal benefit, though they have quite distinct tastes. The root is also edible and commonly used in Thai cuisine.

Cultivation
Sow seeds in spring. An annual, it will grow to 15cm (6in) if regularly picked for leaves, but flower stalks for seed production can reach up to 75cm (2½ft). Coriander can quickly run to seed, which is no problem if that is the intended harvest but irritating if it is the leaves that are desired. Try cultivars such as 'Santo' and 'Leisure' for leaf production.

A History of Healing
Elizabeth Blackwell referred to coriander as being 'frequently used to correct strong purging Medicines', perhaps alluding to its ability to reduce griping, or maybe the propensity of contemporary physicians to over prescribe. It is a gentle aid to digestion, and has been used since ancient times in all herbal traditions against flatulence. Ayurvedic medicine also applies coriander for diabetes, and in the Middle East it is a folk medicine to aid sleep, calming a worrisome mind. European herbals also attribute coriander with aphrodisiac qualities.

Harvesting
Pick leaves as and when required to use fresh. Seeds are ready when they turn papery brown and hard – cut the stems and hang upside down in a paper bag to collect them, then store the seeds in an airtight jar.

How to Use
Add coriander to food, grinding the seeds to a powder and/or scattering fresh leaves over the dish at the last minute. An infused oil of the seeds is said to be beneficial for aching joints and haemorrhoids.

ORIGINS
Northern Europe
and Asia, North
Africa, North
America

CRATAEGUS LAEVIGATA

Hawthorn *May blossom, bread and cheese, haw*

As ancient as it is ubiquitous, hawthorn has been documented as a healing plant since the 1st century BCE. It is associated with pagan and country rituals, such as the choosing of a May Queen, and its flowering branches are said to attract faeries and are considered unlucky when used as a cut flower, especially in churches. *Crataegus laevigata* and *Crataegus monogyna* are very similar plants and can be used interchangeably.

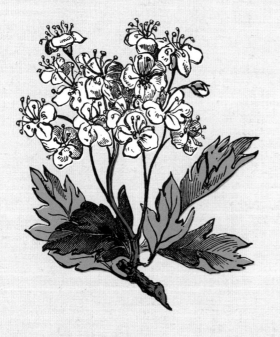

Caution
Consult a qualified herbalist before using hawthorn in the case of cardiovascular conditions.

Cultivation
Although hawthorn makes a pretty garden tree, it is more commonly found in hedgerows both rural and urban. Single, age-old trees can sometimes be seen in the wild, often grown craggy and leaning away from the wind on hillsides and clifftops. Fully hardy, it will survive in all but the poorest soils, in full sun or shade, and withstand the salty blasts of coastal winds.

As a specimen tree it can reach 4–8m (13–26ft) in height and spread, but can also be planted as a productive, pretty but prickly hedge either by itself or in a mixture of other native species. Hawthorn is beloved by wildlife: the leaves are an important food source for the caterpillars of many butterflies and moths, and the berries are vital winter food for birds and small mammals. Pink- and double-flowered varieties are available, but these are neither as efficacious as healing plants nor as attractive to wildlife as the straight species.

A History of Healing

Hawthorn's astringent, diuretic and antioxidant properties give it a wide variety of healing applications. The first mentions of its use are confined to treating kidney and bladder problems: Culpeper wrote that 'The seeds in [the] berries…are held singularly good against the stone.'

A tea of hawthorn leaves and flowers has long been used to calm the flutterings of an anxious heart, and by the end of the 19th-century Western medicine had begun to discover its efficacy in treating heart and circulation diseases. Herbalists continue to use hawthorn preparations to open the blood vessels and strengthen the heart, supported by the results of clinical trials that have proved *Crataegus* extract is helpful when used with other medicines following heart failure.

Both traditional Chinese medicine and Ayurveda apply hawthorn as a means of regulating the body's systems, in particular the blood flow and digestion, but also the memory when combined with *Ginkgo biloba* (see page 115).

Foraging

In mid-spring the hawthorn is covered with blossom – look for it then and make a note of the locations of good bushes/trees so that they are easy to find when the branches are bare of all but berries in late autumn. *Crataegus laevigata* and *C. monogyna* are very similar in appearance to each other and to the many other *Crataegus* species and hybrids, but *C. monogyna* has only a single seed (the species name comes from the Ancient Greek *monos,* meaning 'single', and *gyna* meaning 'seed') within each berry, whereas other species have two seeds.

How to Use

The leaves and/or flowers can be prepared as a tisane (add ginkgo leaves for a memory aid). The leaves can also be eaten raw, added to salads or sandwiches, or chewed by themselves on a hedgerow foraging trip.

To improve the circulation and strengthen the heart, eat the berries (haws). They are more palatable as well as more beneficial for the digestion when cooked, but can be eaten raw for the most benefit to the heart. Haws make a delicious ketchup, or combine them with other hedgerow fruits to make a jelly suitable for sweet or savoury dishes.

A poultice of the leaves and/or fruits is said to be good at drawing out splinters. According to Culpeper: 'And thus you see the thorn does give a medicine for its own pricking.'

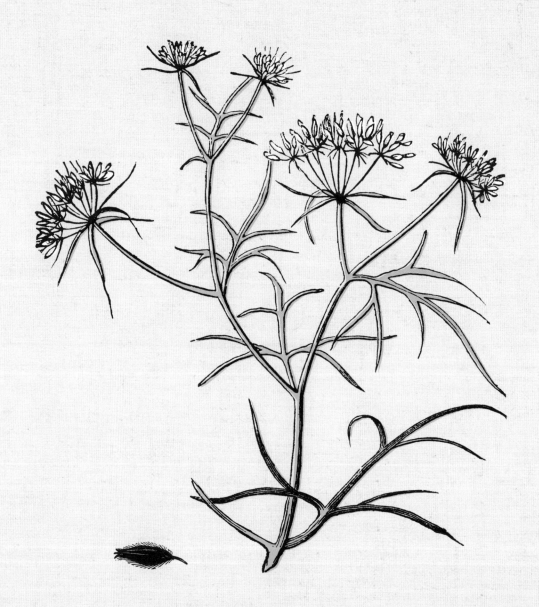

CUMINUM CYMINUM

Cumin *Comino, jeera*

Although used more as a culinary spice today than a therapeutic herb, cumin has an ancient history of medicinal use. It should not be confused with curcumin (turmeric, see page 118) or *Nigella sativa*, commonly called black cumin.

Cultivation

A half-hardy annual, cumin can be sown in spring. Give it a sunny position and well-drained soil with protection from frosts. It will reach around 30cm (12in) in height and spread, but the seed may not ripen without a sufficiently long, hot summer.

A History of Healing

Cumin was popular in Ancient Rome and Greece, and in the latter culture it was considered to symbolize greed and miserliness. It was used in Western medicine as a digestive aid, and in Ayurvedic herbalism to aid the absorption of other herbs. Other Ayurvedic applications include to treat insomnia and, when ground with onion juice, as a remedy for poisonous stings, such as those from scorpions.

Cumin is also one of the herbs mentioned by name in the Bible, with references in Isaiah (28:25, 28:27–8) to cumin being sown and then harvested by threshing the seeds from the stalks: 'Caraway is beaten out with a stick, and cumin with a rod'. It also appears in Matthew 23:23 as being used to pay tithes to the church.

How to Use

Cumin, as with many seeds, is sold in both seed and ground/powdered form. It is always better to grind seeds freshly for their maximum aroma, flavour and potency – a spice grinder is an inexpensive but invaluable piece of equipment, or grind by hand with a pestle and mortar.

Use cumin in cooking, adding it to curries and other sauces, falafel, breads and pickles.

ORIGINS
India

CURCUMA LONGA

Turmeric *Haridra, cucurmin, Jiang Huang*

Perhaps the wonder-herb of the modern age, turmeric is now undergoing extensive research into its healing properties, most of which confirms the traditional herbal uses. Turmeric makes an attractive potted house plant in a well-lit, humid room, such as a bathroom or kitchen, giving large leafy growth and yellow flowers in summer. Widely used as a dye, turmeric will stain yellow anything it comes into contact with, leading to it being used as an adulterant or cheap substitute for mustard and saffron. However, turmeric's smell and taste are quite distinct, as Mrs Grieve noted in her herbal: 'It has a peculiar fragrant odour and a bitterish, slightly acrid, taste, like ginger, exciting warmth in the mouth and colouring the saliva yellow.'

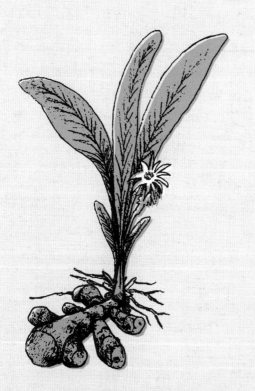

Cultivation

Turmeric reaches around 1m (3ft) tall and can spread indefinitely in the ground. It needs well-drained soil in sun or dappled shade and a minimum temperature of 15°C (59°F). Mist indoor plants once or twice daily to keep a humid atmosphere around the leaves.

A History of Healing

Historically, turmeric was used in both Ayurvedic and traditional Chinese medicine for liver and digestive complaints internally, and externally for skin disorders. In its native India it is thought to slow the aging process.

Modern research has proven turmeric's marked anti-inflammatory properties, and that the black pepper traditionally taken with it does indeed improve the turmeric's absorption. The ability of turmeric to block inflammatory pathways throughout the body makes it a potentially valuable herb to treat arthritis, asthma, eczema, psoriasis, inflammatory bowel disease, stroke and cardiovascular disorders. It is also being investigated for its cholesterol-lowering effects, its potential as an anticancer treatment and its possible benefits in the treatment of Alzheimer's disease.

Harvesting

Lift rhizomes in autumn, and then use them fresh (store in the fridge), or freeze or dry them for future use. Pick the leaves occasionally through the year to wrap around fish or vegetables before cooking, into which they will impart a gentle flavour.

How to Use

Turmeric is best assimilated by the body – therefore making the best use of its active constituents – when consumed with black pepper (see page 186) and preferably some form of fat, such as milk or oil. Add turmeric, fresh or dried, and black pepper to rice, eggs and sauces, or drink it in the form of golden milk (see box).

A paste made from powdered turmeric and honey or water can be applied to the skin for spots or psoriasis, but be warned that it may stain the skin, clothes and bed linen yellow.

GOLDEN MILK

Turmeric lattes are now popular in the West as a health drink, but Ayurvedic medicine has been using a turmeric-infused warm drink for centuries. It is similar to the Malayan drink *teh halia* (ginger tea); both make a warming drink with anti-inflammatory properties.

Pour a large mugful (250–400ml/1–1½ cups) of milk into a saucepan, adding 1 tsp of coconut oil if using a plant-based milk. Add 1 tsp of dried or freshly grated turmeric, a few grinds of black pepper, 1 tsp of freshly grated ginger, 2–3 cardamom pods and a cinnamon stick (use other flavourings, if preferred). Bring to a very gentle simmer for 10 minutes. Strain into a mug and stir in honey to taste.

CYMBOPOGON CITRATUS

Lemon grass

The long leaves of lemon grass are full of the essential oils citral and citronellal, which are important economically for their use in perfumery, aromatherapy and food flavourings. These volatile oils make lemon grass plants effective insect repellents in summertime, but they are also attractive to cats, who like to bat (and inadvertently shred) the leaves.

Cultivation

A tropical grass reaching up to 1m (3ft) in height and spread, lemon grass needs a minimum temperature of 7°C (45°F), well-drained soil and a sunny position. In a temperate climate, grow as a potted house plant, moving it outside for the summer once it is warm enough. Inside, mist regularly to maintain humidity.

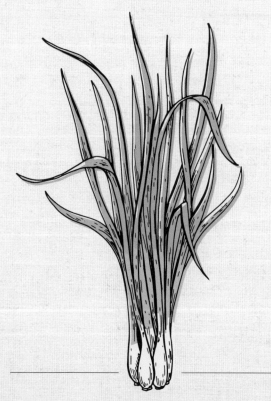

A History of Healing

The traditional uses of lemon grass centre around its reputation as a tonic to relax and soothe minor digestive complaints, and it is often used for children for whom other herbs would be too potent. It is also applied to reduce fevers, especially in Caribbean folk medicine. Externally, the leaves are used as a poultice or paste to treat ringworm, and the diluted essential oil is massaged into painful arthritic joints.

In Tanzania, the flowers of the related species *C. densiflorus* are smoked by medicine men, who believe they will then experience prophetic dreams.

Tips for Growing

Lemon grass will often root from a fresh stem bought in the shops. Choose a healthy stem, and put into a glass with enough water to cover the base. Leave on a sunny windowsill until the stem sprouts roots – this could take several weeks – changing the water periodically. Pot up the sprouted stem and grow on.

How to Use

Infuse fresh leaves into hot water for a delicious, relaxing tea. Dried leaves have a more bitter, inferior taste, so keep a plant on the windowsill for a permanent supply of fresh leaves.

CYNARA SCOLYMUS

Globe artichoke

Artichokes, and their cousins the cardoon, make stately additions to the veg patch or flower border, but even artichoke heads bought at the market can have a beneficial herbal effect.

Caution
Artichokes belong to the Asteraceae family and should be avoided by anyone with allergies to these plants.

Cultivation
Artichokes can reach 2m (6½ft) tall and over 1m (3ft) wide, so allow them plenty of space to grow and perhaps some form of supporting cage in windy spots. They thrive in rich, well-drained soil in full sun. Growing from seed offers the greatest range of varieties, which therapeutically are interchangeable.

A History of Healing
Dioscorides wrote that the mashed root of artichokes when applied to the armpits or other parts of the body would sweeten unpleasant body odours. Culpeper had an even more intimate suggestion, which he attributed to artichokes being 'under the dominion of Venus': 'It is no marvel that they [therefore] provoke lust... and yet they stay the involuntary course of natural seed in man, which is commonly called nocturnal pollutions.'

Artichokes are also greatly valued, especially on the European continent, as a food. All parts of the plant when eaten or drunk as an infusion are bitter and therefore benefit the digestion. Artichokes support liver function and are particularly good at stimulating the production of bile, necessary for breaking down fats during digestion, which in turn results in better vitamin absorption. Several trials have also shown that artichokes lower fats in the blood.

Harvesting
Pick young leaves in spring, before the flower buds appear, to use fresh or to dry. Cut the flower heads before the side bracts open.

How to Use
Infuse the leaves in hot water for a digestive and liver stimulant; add other herbs or honey to temper the bitterness, if liked. Artichokes contain a compound, cynarin, which once consumed will make subsequent foods or drinks taste sweeter. When boiling artichokes to eat, the cooking water can also be drunk as a tea.

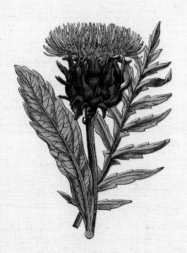

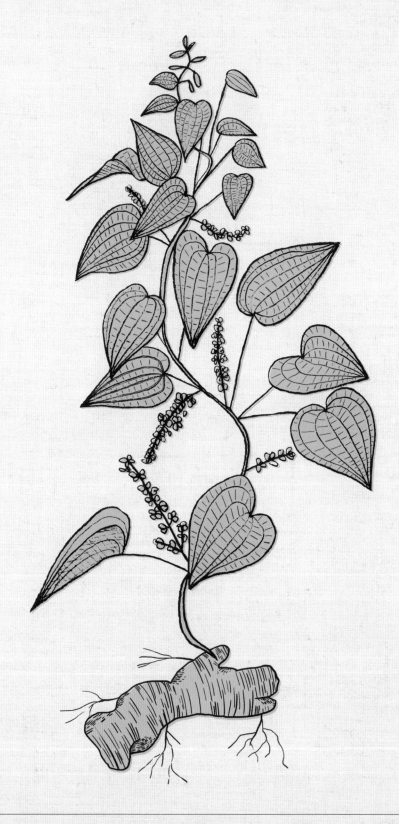

DIOSCOREA VILLOSA

Wild yam *Colic root, rheumatism root*

Wild yam's secondary common names date from the time European settlers
arrived in the Americas and began to use the root for both colic and rheumatism.
However, the discovery of its steroidal compounds in the 20th century have been
the plant's main contribution to medical history.

Caution
Contraindicated during pregnancy.

Cultivation
A fully hardy, deciduous perennial climber,
wild yam grows to around 5m (16½ft) tall.
It prefers rich, well-drained soil in full sun
or partial shade.

A History of Healing
Traditionally, wild yam was used to ease the pain
and inflammation of digestive conditions and
menstrual problems. It is a bitter herb, and in
traditional Chinese medicine it is valued as a
tonic for the digestion.

Wild yams contain substances called
saponins, which are used in the manufacture
of pharmaceutical steroids. Their effects on the
hormones have long been known, as wild yam
is a traditional remedy in its native Central
America for menstrual and labour pains, but
in the mid-20th century isolated compounds
from wild yam were the origin of the first
contraceptive pill. Until synthetic alternatives
were found in the 1970s, yam crops (of a
related species) were the only source of these
steroids for the pill.

Harvesting
Dig up part of the rhizomes (roots) in autumn
and dry before using.

How to Use
A decoction of the rhizomes (roots) is thought
to be beneficial for irritable bowel syndrome
and other inflammatory conditions.

ECHINACEA

Echinacaea *Coneflower*

Echinacea's name is variously described as being inspired by either the
Ancient Greek for hedgehog, *ekhinos*, or the Latin for sea urchin, *echinus*.
The description is apt in either way: the flower's bristly central cone is more
prominent than the reflexed purple petals that surround it. It is a valuable
flower for pollinators and makes a pretty cut flower. *E. purpurea*, *E. angustifolia*
and *E. pallida* can all be used interchangeably. *E. purpurea* was adopted as the
main crop in Europe when the seed of *E. angustifolia* became scarce and, proving
easier to cultivate, *E. purpurea* continues to be most widely grown today.

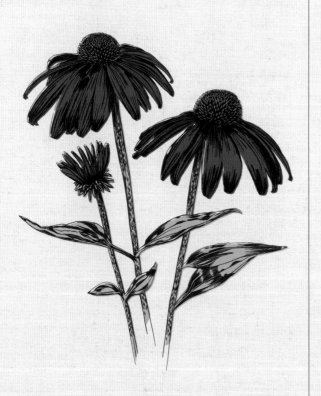

Caution
**In cases of autoimmune conditions, seek
professional medical advice before using
echinacea, as it may interact with prescribed
medication and/or cause a flare-up of the
disease. Echinacea is a member of the
Asteraceae family and should be avoided by
anyone with allergies to these plants.**

Cultivation
This hardy herbaceous perennial will thrive
in full sun and a rich, well-drained soil. The
different species will reach around 1–1.5m
(3–5ft) in height and 40–60cm (16–24in)
in spread.

A History of Healing

Used by Native American tribes to treat both internal and external infections (including snake bites), echinacea has a lasting reputation as a powerful herbal plant. Today, it is possibly the most well known of herbal preparations for colds and flu, yet research has still not exactly proven what makes it so effective. It contains a number of active constituents, and it seems these work best synergistically rather than when isolated.

Herbalists advise taking echinacea to benefit the immune system, both as a preventative and as a treatment, promoting a speedy recovery and also supporting the body through post-viral and chronic fatigue. It works by stimulating the production of white blood cells, making it useful against both bacterial and viral infections. It has a long history of particularly effective action against sore throats.

Applied externally, echinacea has been reputed to reduce the effects of aging and UV damage to the skin, and to help heal skin infections and wounds, including conditions such as psoriasis and acne.

Foraging and Buying

All three main species of echinacea are endangered in the wild in their native habitat, so do not forage for wild plants, and ensure that roots and preparations bought from herbal suppliers are sourced from commercially grown plants.

How to Use

Roots and rhizomes lifted in autumn can be dried to use throughout the year. The best-quality roots have a tingling sensation when placed on the tongue. Prepare the root as a decoction or tincture to support the immune system and benefit skin conditions such as cold sores and chronic disorders. Powdered root in capsule form and tinctures are also available to buy over the counter. For sore throats, gargle with the decoction or prepare the recipe below, which will store for a year, to be taken as needed.

SORE THROAT GARGLE

Wilt a handful of sage for 24 hours in a warm place. Place the sage in a large glass jar with around 50g (2 tbsp) of dried echinacea root, 1 tbsp of dried or fresh elderberries and a pinch of whole cloves. Cover with around 200ml (¾ cup) vodka and seal. Leave to infuse, shaking daily, for two weeks before straining and bottling. To use, dilute a spoonful in a small cup of boiled and cooled water (add a spoonful of honey for an added antiseptic and soothing benefit) and gargle, swallowing or spitting out, as desired.

ELETTARIA CARDAMOMUM

Cardamom *Ela, elettari*

Good-quality cardamom has a eucalyptus-type scent, while inferior pods are more camphoric. The seeds are widely used in Scandinavian baking, and as an ingredient of relaxing chai tea. Cardamom essential oil is also important in perfumery, especially for eau de cologne and aftershave.

Cultivation

Cardamom's aromatic foliage makes it an attractive house plant for temperate climates – give it a rich potting compost and dappled shade. In the wild, this perennial reaches a height and spread of 3m (10ft) and needs a minimum temperature of 10°C (50°F).

A History of Healing

Ayurvedic medicine uses cardamom for digestive and bronchial complaints. By the 4th century BCE it was known and valued in Greece, exported along the caravan routes that ran from

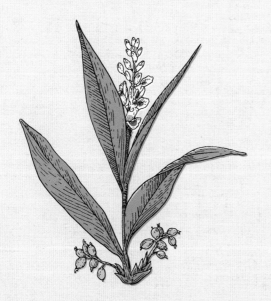

East to West and back again, but it was not recorded as a medicinal plant in China until the 8th century CE, as a remedy for urinary incontinence.

Cardamom is a reputed aphrodisiac, yet it is also widely used as a relaxing and sleep-inducing herb, which perhaps explains the traditional Arabic combination of adding cardamom to coffee.

Tips for Buying

Buy cardamom still in the seedpod, and always grind seeds freshly from the pod because cardamom quickly loses much of its aroma once ground. Good-quality pods will be green in colour.

How to Use

Infuse the pods whole into sweet and savoury dishes, or grind the seeds to use in baking, such as cardamom buns. Alternatively, crush two to three pods and infuse the pods and seeds in hot water to make a refreshing after-dinner drink, to benefit the digestion and sweeten the breath. Infuse in equal parts milk and water with other spices such as cinnamon, ginger, nutmeg and tea – use personal favourites – to make a delicious chai tea. The essential oil can be mixed with a carrier oil and massaged into the abdomen for bloating and other digestive pain.

ORIGINS
Europe, North
Asia, North Africa,
Americas

EQUISETUM ARVENSE

Horsetail *Bottlebrush, shave grass, field horsetail*

Few gardeners would actively choose to cultivate horsetail, a plant
so pervasive and strong it has survived since the Palaeozoic era and is
now considered a dreadful weed that is almost impossible to eradicate.
However, scanty use of it as a therapeutic herb can go a little way to
forgiving it in the hearts of gardeners.

Caution
**Avoid during pregnancy and in cases
of heart or kidney conditions. Exercise
caution handling dried material – the dust
is a particular lung irritant. Horsetail can
inhibit the body's use of vitamin B: avoid
in cases of low levels, supplement horsetail
remedies with a vitamin B tablet and do not
take for extended periods.**

Cultivation
Horsetail spreads by means of spores produced
under ground and by its fleshy white roots,
which descend sideways and deep into the soil
and easily break when removal is attempted.
Shoots appear in spring, at first resembling
slender asparagus and then sprouting side
growth, making them look like bottlebrushes – it
is these that can be harvested for herbal use.

A History of Healing
Horsetail is an excellent battlefield herb, quickly
staunching both internal and external bleeding
and promoting healing of the tissues: 'It is very
powerfull to staunch bleedings…eyther inward
or outward, the juice or decoction thereof being
drunke, or…applied outwardly' and it 'soon
sodereth together [fuses together] the toppes
of greene wounds,' wrote Parkinson. It is now
known these effects are due to horsetail's high
silica content, which also makes it beneficial
for healing and strengthening the bones, skin,
hair and nails, as well as scouring dirty pots, its
traditional use.

How to Use
Horsetail is best used sparingly and sporadically,
when the body needs strengthening perhaps
after injury or long illness. The plant can be
juiced or infused into hot water, a syrup or
tincture; pair it with a demulcent herb such as
marsh mallow to lessen its irritant effect. It can
also be added to a herbal bath.

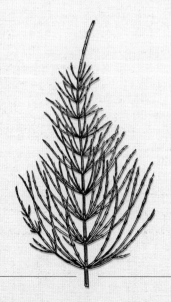

ORIGINS
North America
(*Eschscholzia*) Europe,
Asia, North Africa
(*Papaver*)

ESCHSCHOLZIA CALIFORNICA | *PAPAVER*

Californian poppy and poppy

All poppies have some sedative effect, despite being distinct species. The most potent is the opium poppy (*Papaver somniferum*) which is subject to cultivation restrictions, but other species are easily grown and have healing benefits.

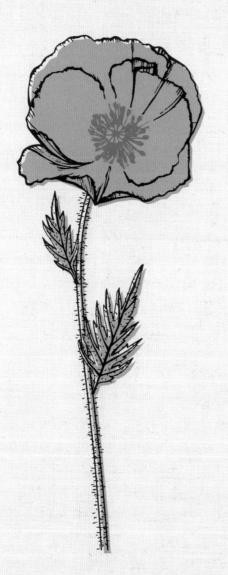

Cultivation

Both *Eschscholzia* and *Papaver* poppies are fully hardy, prefer well-drained soil in full sun, and will happily self-seed around the garden, including into paving cracks and gravel paths. It 'springs again of its own sowing', wrote Culpeper. In a normal soil they will reach 60cm (2ft) high and 30cm (12in) wide, but less if growing in poorer conditions.

A History of Healing

The state flower of California, *Eschscholzia* is mildly sedative without the addictive and damaging side-effects of the opium poppy. Native Americans chewed the leaves for their sap, particularly for toothache, and both the leaves and seeds were used by early settlers to aid sleep, especially in children. In Europe the corn poppy (*Papaver rhoeas*) was used in a similar way. Culpeper also wrote that, 'The garden Poppy heads with seeds made into a syrup, is frequently, and to good effect used to procure rest, and sleep, in the sick and weak' and that the leaves were 'also put into hollow teeth, to ease the pain.'

Harvesting

Poppy seedheads of all species are revealed when the petals fall. They then begin to ripen and dry out, eventually revealing small gaps just under the flat, daisy-shaped top. When the stalk sways in the breeze, the seeds are shaken out onto the ground. To ensure a decent harvest, cut the stems as soon as the holes appear and tie them into a paper bag. Hang upside down in a cool, dry place to dry fully, then shake out and store the seeds.

How to Use

Poppy seeds from either *E. californica* or *P. rhoeas* can be sprinkled over food or used in baking. They can also be infused in hot water, as can the leaves and flowers of *E. californica*, and, combined with other restful herbs, make a relaxing bedtime drink. For a tickly sore throat, mash ½ teaspoon of seeds with ½ teaspoon of honey and take just before going to bed – the honey will coat the throat while the seeds impart a mild analgesic effect.

POPPIES FOR POETS AND SOLDIERS

Papaver somniferum, the opium poppy, is the species from which opium and its derivatives laudanum and morphine are taken, and plants have been grown for their sedative properties for around 7,000 years. Today, it is well known for its addictive, highly damaging effects on the body and it is illegal to cultivate without a licence in many countries. Opium was equally notorious in 18th- and 19th-century Europe, when it was the drug of choice for many artistic souls who immortalized its effects in prose and poetry, and it had a similar level of recreational as well as medicinal use in China.

Papaver rhoeas (red, corn, common or Flanders poppy) is similarly sedative, yet has a far milder effect than the opium poppy that makes its seeds safe to eat. Once a common sight in wheat fields, they would adorn the hat of the 'Harvest Lord', denoting him as the man in charge of the labourers bringing home the harvest. Poppy plants produce hundreds of seeds each, which are shaken out of the seedhead when ripe, scattering on the ground either to germinate the following year or become buried by the plough, remaining there sometimes for decades. Churning up the soil brings long-buried seeds to the surface where they can at last flower: when the farmland of Northern Europe was torn up by the trenches and artillery blasts of the First World War, poppies grew in their thousands. The poppy is now a symbol of remembrance for soldiers lost in all wars.

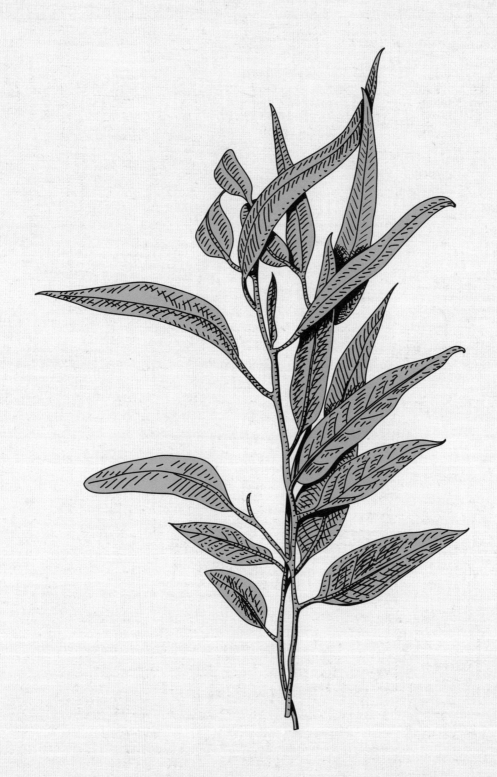

ORIGINS
Australia

EUCALYPTUS GLOBULUS

Eucalyptus *Blue gum*

Eucalyptus are fast-growing trees, although easily coppiced; their timber
is particularly good and was used for the keels of ships in the 19th century.
The trees use a vast volume of water, and so can inhibit the growth of other
species, but on the other hand are excellent at drying marshy ground. Planted
deliberately in this way they not only provide a useful harvest but also reduce
the incidence of mosquitos and malaria.

Caution
**Contraindicated during pregnancy and for
young children. Do not apply undiluted
essential oil to the skin.**

Cultivation
Eucalyptus trees can grow to 30–40m (100–130ft)
tall, and while regular pruning will keep the
branches and trunk to size, if desired, the roots
can spread widely, so allow them plenty of space.
They are frost hardy but will not withstand
severe or prolonged cold weather.

A History of Healing
The traditional Aboriginal remedy for a wide
range of cold and flu symptoms is now popular
worldwide as a natural remedy, and it forms
part of many over-the-counter medicines.
It acts as an expectorant, helping to shift chest
infections and catarrh, and is also antiseptic,
which makes it effective against sore throats
and other infections.

Harvesting
Other eucalyptus can be used in place of
E. globulus, although some have oils that are more
fragranced than medicinally useful. Pick the
adult leaves to use fresh at any time of year.

How to Use
Add a few leaves or drops of essential oil to a
bath or steaming bowl (see page 54) to help
decongest during a cold. To the same end,
essential oil diluted with a carrier oil can be
massaged into the chest. Eucalyptus leaves can
be infused in hot water or other hot drinks,
such as elderberry syrup (see page 213).

FILIPENDULA ULMARIA

Meadowsweet *Queen of the meadow, bridewort*

A wonderfully fragrant herb, meadowsweet is easily foraged for its almond-scented frothy flowers; according to Gerard, 'the smell thereof...[does] delighteth the senses'.

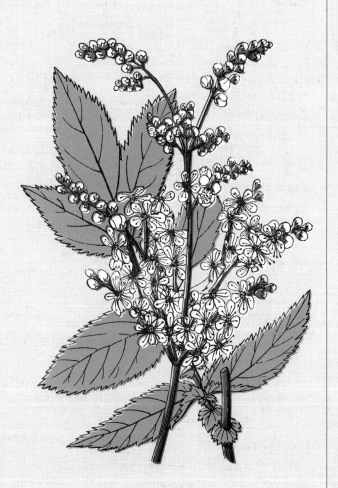

Caution
Contraindicated for anyone with allergies to aspirin, and during pregnancy or breastfeeding.

Cultivation
Rich, damp to boggy soil in full sun or partial shade will suit meadowsweet best. It can reach 1.5m (5ft) tall and 60cm (2ft) wide. Cut back the old growth of this hardy perennial in late winter.

A History of Healing
Culpeper wrote that meadowsweet was said 'to make a merry heart', and Parkinson claimed it was a favourite of Queen Elizabeth I, 'who did more desire it than any other sweet herbe to strew her Chambers withall'. Meadowsweet was also traditionally used to flavour mead and beer – its name derives from 'mead-wort' (mead-herb) – and it was a sacred herb of the Druids. It is a traditional country-wedding flower.

However, meadowsweet's most significant contribution to medicine is as the origin of aspirin, the name of which derives from the plant's old botanical name, *Spiraea*. It contains compounds called salicylates, which were first isolated from meadowsweet in 1836 (and are also found in willow, see page 204), and then synthesized as aspirin in 1899. Aspirin is an anti-inflammatory and analgesic drug, but can be highly irritant to the digestive tract; meadowsweet has a synergistic effect whereby the rest of the plant protects and heals the body as well as providing pain relief.

Foraging

Meadowsweet is in flower for most of the summer and grows on the banks of rivers and streams. Hang whole stems and pick the flowers off once dry.

How to Use

The almond/elderflower flavour and fragrance of the flowers make them a useful culinary herb for infusing into creamy puddings and sorbets; they can be substituted into any recipe that calls for elderflowers, including the cordial recipe below. For a mild painkiller and/or to soothe the digestion or arthritis, drink cordial diluted over ice or diluted in hot water, or infuse the flowers directly in hot or cold water. The flowers can also be added to baths.

MEADOWSWEET (OR ELDERFLOWER) CORDIAL

This basic cordial recipe can be adapted for almost any herb, such as lemon balm or mint, to make a refreshing and therapeutic summer drink or a warming and soothing winter one. Leafy herbs can be added in sprigs. Flowers should be picked in daylight when fully open and should be separated from the stems (especially elderflowers, as the stems are mildly toxic) – leave them to dry for a few hours after picking then crumble the flowers off the stalks.

1kg (5 cups) unrefined golden caster sugar

1.4 litres (2½ pints) water

20–25 meadowsweet flower heads (or a large bowlful of herb flowers or leafy sprigs)

zest and juice of 2 lemons

Mix the sugar and water in a large saucepan over a gentle heat, stirring until the sugar is completely dissolved. Bring to the boil, then simmer for 20 minutes, or until thickened slightly. Take the pan off the heat and stir in the herbs and lemon zest and juice. Cover with a lid and leave for 24 hours, stirring occasionally. Strain out the herbs and pour into sterilized bottles, seal and label.

It will keep for 6 months unopened in the fridge – use within 1–2 weeks once opened. Frozen, it will keep for one year – use plastic bottles or freeze in ice-cube trays then pop out and store in a sealed and labelled bag or box in the freezer.

FOENICULUM VULGARE

Fennel *Wild fennel*

Most herbals concern themselves with fennel rather than its vegetable counterpart Florence/sweet fennel, as the latter is considered less therapeutically potent. Giant fennel (*Ferula communis*) is a different and extremely poisonous species.

Caution
Contraindicated during pregnancy.

Cultivation
Fennel is a hardy perennial which should be planted in light, well-drained soil in full sun. Cut back the old growth in late winter. It reaches 2m (6½ft) tall and 50cm (20in) wide.

A History of Healing
Fennel has been used since ancient times as a digestive aid. The 'Nine Herbs Prayer' from the Anglo-Saxon herbal text *Lacnunga* describes fennel as 'very mighty'. The plant also has a long-standing use as an eyewash to treat infections; Dioscorides wrote that 'the juice, when put into the eye, aids vision'. Culpeper mentioned this, too, as well as its ability to increase the flow of breast milk in nursing mothers. He also wrote that the 'leaves, seeds, and roots thereof are much used in drink or broth, to make people more lean that are too fat.'

How to Use
Infuse the seeds in hot water to soothe the digestion and alleviate bloating; crush the seeds first to release the oils more effectively. Do not take fennel seeds to excess, as they can be toxic in large amounts. A teaspoon only of cooled infusions can be given to children in the case of tummy upsets.

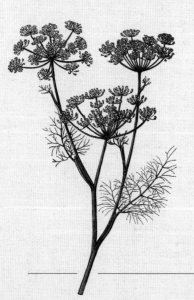

HEALING HERBAL SALADS

There are far more interesting and flavourful leaves to put into a salad than just lettuce! The more variety in our diet, the better, so try adding some of the herb leaves below. When picking, be aware that the older the leaf, the tougher and more bitter it will be.

• basil • chickweed • coriander • dandelion • dill • fennel • lemon balm
• mint • nasturtium • parsley • yarrow

Perhaps include a few herbal flowers, too:
• cornflower • borage • marigold • nasturtium

ORIGINS
Europe, North
and West Asia

GALIUM APARINE

Cleavers *Sticky willy, goosegrass*

Infusions of cleavers have a pleasant verdant, cucumber-like flavour. Related species to cleavers include sweet woodruff (*G. odoratum*), which is added to wine and fruit cups, including the traditional German spring drink *Maibowle*, and *Galium verum*, historically used for curdling and colouring cheese. *Galium* derives from the Greek *gala*, meaning 'milk'.

Cultivation

A common garden weed and hedgerow plant, cleavers prefer slightly damp soil and partial shade. The stems straggle and flop over the top of other plants, with no definite height or spread. Hardy annuals, they spread via their sticky seeds.

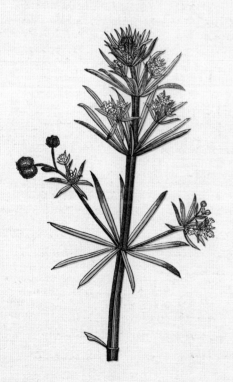

A History of Healing

Cleavers are primarily associated with detoxifying. Taken internally as a juice or an infusion, they have been used since ancient times to cleanse and purify, with Dioscorides recommending the plant for combatting weariness, and modern herbalists for chronic fatigue syndrome and glandular fever. This diuretic and cleansing action has also resulted in their use to alleviate symptoms of skin disorders, from scrofula to psoriasis, either taken internally or applied externally as a poultice. An old saying about cleavers goes along the lines of, 'Whosoever shall drink cleavers water for nine weeks shall have the skin of an angel.'

How to Use

Use cleavers as a seasonal spring tonic; by late spring, the tiny hairs on the plant make it less palatable and it is not easy to dry. Culpeper wrote, 'It is a good remedy in the Spring...to keep the body in health, and fitting it for that change of season that is coming.' The stems can also be mashed and frozen in an ice-cube tray, where they will last a further couple of months. Infuse a good handful of cleavers in around 250ml (1 cup) of cold water overnight, adding a slice of lemon, orange or ginger for more flavour, and drink the following day.

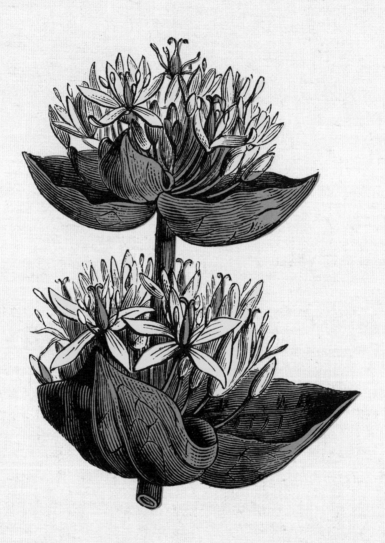

ORIGINS
Mountainous
regions across
Southern Europe

GENTIANA LUTEA

Gentian *Yellow gentian, bitterwort*

Gentian is probably the most bitter substance known to man, with its bitter compounds still detectable on the palate even at dilutions of 1:12,000. As such, it is a classic digestive bitter and a principal ingredient in some traditional aperitifs and bitters, such as Angostura bitters.

Caution
Do not use in the case of gastric or duodenal ulcers.

Cultivation
A hardy perennial, gentian will grow in full sun or partial shade and in most well-drained soils; prolonged time in wet soil can cause root rot. It will reach 1–2m (3–6½ft) tall, depending on conditions, with a spread of around 60cm (2ft).

A History of Healing
King Gentius of Illyria discovered the benefits of the plant in c.500 BCE, and so gave it his name. Since then it has been used as an all-round digestive tonic, stimulating the appetite and improving the general functioning of the digestive system. Current research is now investigating these properties to prove gentian's potential as a treatment for inflammation in the gut and also as a possible anticancer drug.

Culpeper used his entry on gentian to point out the advantages of using home-grown herbs rather than importing them, and encouraging his readers to seek out local plant remedies: '[Gentian] is brought over from beyond sea, yet we have two sorts of it growing frequently in our nation, which, besides the reasons so frequently alleged why English herbs should be fittest for English bodies, has been proved by the experience of divers physicians, to be not a wit inferior in virtue to that which comes from beyond sea.'

Harvesting
Dig up a part of the rhizomes (roots) in autumn and dry before using.

How to Use
Roots can be prepared as a decoction or tincture and taken in small quantities before a meal.

GINKGO BILOBA

Ginkgo *Maidenhair tree, Bai Guo*

Ginkgo is the oldest living tree species and often referred to as a living fossil; the DNA of ginkgo trees growing today is indistinguishable from fossilized specimens dating back 270 million years. Botanically it is unique: it is the only member of its genus, the only seed-bearing plant to have fan-shaped leaves with veins radiating out to the edges, and while it is usually grouped with conifers and cycads, it is actually neither, having its own class, Ginkgoopsida. It makes a striking specimen tree, columnar in shape with brilliant yellow autumn foliage.

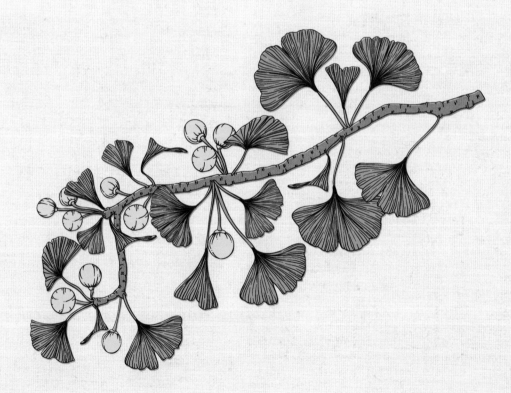

Caution

Ginkgo can be toxic in excess. Do not take ginkgo with blood-thinning medication. Some countries restrict its use.

Cultivation

Ginkgo trees can reach 40m (130ft) tall and 8m (26ft) wide, but will take up to 50 years to do so. The trees are deciduous and fully hardy. For fruit and seed production, both a female and male tree are needed, and successful pollination and fruit development require a warm summer. Plant in fertile, well-drained soil in full sun and do not prune, as this can cause dieback.

A History of Healing

Traditional Chinese medicine has been prescribing ginkgo since 2800 BCE for asthma and coughs. The plant has both anti-inflammatory and anti-allergenic properties, and herbalists today still recommend it as a remedy for asthma. Modern research has shown that ginkgo contains unique compounds (called ginkgolides) which inhibit the body's allergic responses and may have a protective effect on nerve cells.

Ginkgo is also widely used as a stimulant to the circulation, especially to the brain, and it is considered good for the memory. It is a popular tonic in China and mainland Europe for maintaining cognitive function into old age and aiding recovery after a stroke. Clinical studies on the effects of ginkgo in these fields and as a possible treatment for dementia and Alzheimer's disease have had mixed results, possibly due to varying levels of the active constituents in the extracts used in the trials. Ginkgo is also being investigated for its potential in alleviating the symptoms of depression.

Harvesting

Pick the leaves as they begin to turn yellow in autumn, and use fresh or dried. The unpleasant-smelling fruits yield a single seed each, which can be dried and then roasted to add to soups, stir-fries and other dishes, or eaten as a snack.

How to Use

Infuse the leaves in hot water for a warming drink to help strengthen the circulation, especially in the case of cold hands and feet and/or varicose veins (combine it with hawthorn, see page 114). Ginkgo tea can also help the memory and concentration.

GLYCYRRHIZA GLABRA

Liquorice

Liquorice has been cultivated in the UK since the Middle Ages, and known there for much longer: it was sufficiently popular by 1305 for Edward I to tax liquorice imports to raise money for the building of London Bridge. It crops up in all the medieval herbals as well as inventories such as the 1264 accounts of King Henry IV, but is most commonly associated with the Yorkshire town of Pontefract. Dominican friars in the monastery there began to cultivate liquorice on a large scale, and liquorice pastilles are still known as pomfrets, a corruption of Pontefract cakes, today.

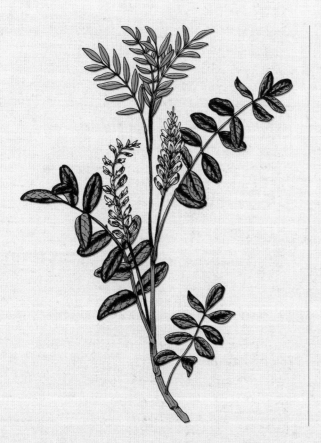

Liquorice means sweet-root and although the glycyrrhizin it contains is 50 times sweeter than sugar, liquorice is far less harmful to health than sucrose. It is used as a flavouring in many foods and drinks, notably various confectionary such as Liquorice Allsorts and the island of Jersey preserve Black Butter, and to give stout its dark colouring.

Caution
Contraindicated with blood pressure
medication; long-term use at high doses
can raise blood pressure. Not advised
during pregnancy.

Cultivation

Liquorice grows best in full sun and a light, sandy soil from which the roots are more easily accessed. A hardy perennial, it can reach 1.5m (5ft) tall and 1m (3ft) wide. It is an attractive plant with pinnate leaves and loose spikes of violet pea-like flowers, but once planted it is difficult to eradicate.

A History of Healing

A demulcent herb, liquorice has been used for bronchial complaints such as coughs, sore throats and asthma since ancient times. It was, and still is, also used to treat mouth ulcers and ulcers of the stomach, especially in the case of acid reflux, coating the tissues and soothing inflammation. Various trials have shown it to be effective in protecting the liver and in the treatment of hepatitis C. The drug carbenoxolene (now superseded), used to treat stomach ulcers in the 1960s, was developed from glycyrrizin extracted from liquorice.

Glycyrrhizin, once broken down in the gut, has a similar anti-inflammatory effect to corticosteroid hormones such as hydrocortisone, and it stimulates hormone production in the adrenal glands. Overall, liquorice can have an adaptogenic tonic effect, supporting the adrenal glands, particularly during stressful periods. Another compound of liquorice is known to be oestrogenic, so it is also used by herbalists to treat hot flushes and other menopausal symptoms.

Parkinson, as well as detailing liquorice's various remedial actions, wrote that it can be made into a beer-like drink, which would become alcoholic if left to ferment with yeast: 'Licoris boiled in water, with a little Cinnamon added to it, serveth instead of drinke in many places, especially if it be set to work with barme [a brewer's yeast-type substance] as beere is.'

Harvesting

On three- to four-year-old plants, unearth the roots on one side. There will be two forms – a taproot growing downwards, and horizontal rhizomes growing out from it. Cut off the horizontal growth but leave the taproot, and harvest from the opposite side the following year. Dry the roots before using.

How to Use

Liquorice is a wonderful sugar-free sweetener for herbal teas, as well as a remedy in its own right, to support hormonal balance and relieve digestive discomfort or coughs and colds. It pairs particularly well with mint, or take a lead from Parkinson and infuse it with cinnamon. Liquorice sticks, made from the dried juice, can be chewed for an occasional herbal sweet.

HAMAMELIS VIRGINIANA

Witch hazel

Apparently witch hazel's benefits to health were sealed among ancient European physicians when it was decided that the curling tendrils of the flowers represented the snake coiling around the staff of Asclepius, the Greek god of medicine. This may be fanciful, but modern research has now proven the effectiveness of witch hazel treatments for the skin and it is widely available in pharmacies as a distillation.

Caution
Use externally only and do not apply to broken skin.

Cultivation
Hardy witch hazel forms a large shrub with spreading branches, reaching 5m (16½ft) by 4m (13ft). Plant in moist, rich soil in full sun or partial shade.

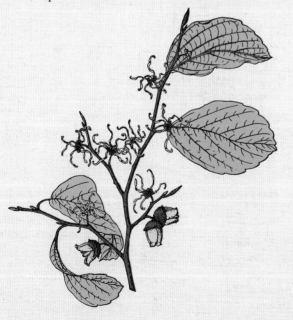

A History of Healing
European settlers in America learned about witch hazel from the indigenous tribespeople, and saw how effective it was in treating bruising, skin sores and inflamed skin. It is powerfully astringent, and is therefore applied to any skin condition in which a tightening effect is needed, such as varicose veins, greasy or spotty skin, bruising and hot, swollen legs in summer. A number of studies have proven it as a particularly effective natural remedy for haemorrhoids, as well as healing for external rashes such as nappy rash.

Harvesting
Cut young twigs once the plant is in full leaf in spring and use fresh or dry.

How to Use
Witch hazel can be prepared as a decoction that can be stored in the fridge – it will keep for around a week; discard any mouldy preparations – and used as a cooling spray in hot weather.

HIBISCUS SABDARIFFA

Hibiscus *Jamaica sorrel, roselle, karkadé*

All hibiscus, including *Hibiscus rosa-sinensis*, the most common garden and conservatory hibiscus, and also the annual *H. trionum*, which is grown at the Chelsea Physic Garden, have herbal properties and are also used as a pictorial trope for tropical or exotic countries.

Cultivation

Hibiscus need well-drained but moist soil in full sun – they will not flower well in poor summers – and a minimum temperature of 10°C (50°F). Plants can reach 2.5m (8ft) tall and 2m (6½ft) wide, but can be cut back hard in spring.

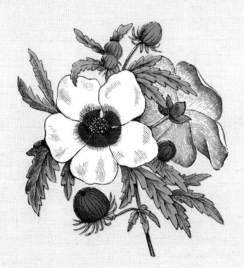

A History of Healing

The bright red calyces (the part of the flower surrounding the petals) of the hibiscus are used as a colourant and flavouring in many proprietary herbal and fruit tea blends, but the teas were initially unpopular when first brought to Europe in the 19th century because of that very colour! The flowers are sacred to the god Ganesh and valued in Hindu ceremonies. Hibiscus means 'plant that is consecrated to the ibis', a sacred bird in ancient Egypt.

Hibiscus infusions have a generalized tonic effect. They are rich in vitamin C, and studies have shown the calyces to have a significant anti-oxidant effect and may help lower blood pressure.

How to Use

Add hibiscus flowers or dried calyces to herbal teas as a general tonic and flavouring.

HUMULUS LUPULUS

Hop

A bough of hops hung over the hearth is an attractive, if musty-smelling, decoration that is said to bring good luck for the following twelvemonth, provided it is replaced fresh each harvest.

Caution
Contraindicated during pregnancy and breastfeeding and for young children. Hops should not be taken internally over long periods or in the case of depression.

Cultivation
Hops are an extremely vigorous hardy perennial climber; the variety 'Prima Donna' is relatively dwarfed, while 'Aureus' has golden yellow leaves. Plant in moist soil in full sun or partial shade. The flower cones are poisonous to dogs and cats, so exercise caution when planting them. Cut back the previous year's growth in late winter.

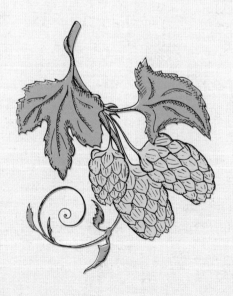

A History of Healing
Although now inextricably linked with the making of beer, hops were slow to be accepted as an alternative bitter herb for brewing, and indeed were actually outlawed as a flavouring by both Henry VI and Henry VIII. Herbally, they were generally used as a digestive tonic – Culpeper recommended them mostly for cleansing and purging – although it is said that George III was prescribed a hop pillow to help ease his supposed madness.

Native American tribes traditionally used hops for calming frayed nerves and alleviating insomnia and pain. This sedative effect is still the main herbal use of hops today, either taken internally or when the fragrance is inhaled. This effect is supported by evidence from clinical studies.

Harvesting
Pick the cone-shaped flowers when they are sticky and green, before they brown at the edges.

How to Use
Infuse dried hops in hot water, perhaps with chamomile or a lemony herb, for an occasional bedtime drink, to ease restlessness and encourage sleep. A safer long-term use is to place the dried flowers in a cotton sachet, with lavender, if liked, to tuck under the pillow.

HYDRASTIS CANADENSIS

Goldenseal *Orangeroot, yellowroot*

Goldenseal was so highly prized as a panacea in 19th-century America that wild populations of it became massively depleted, leading to the authorities declaring it an endangered species in 1997.

Caution
Contraindicated during pregnancy, for children and for people with high blood pressure. Toxic if taken to excess. Inhibits vitamin B absorption if taken in the long term.

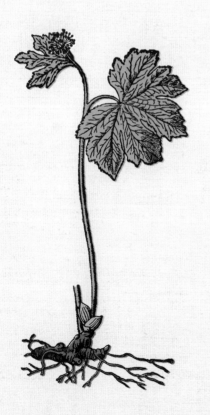

Cultivation
Goldenseal prefers moist, rich but not boggy soil in shade. A hardy perennial, it will grow to 30cm (12in) tall and around 20cm (8in) wide.

A History of Healing
Some herbs garner a reputation as a cure-all, and so it was for goldenseal. Used as an insect repellent (when ground with bear fat) and a salve for eye complaints, wounds and digestive problems by the Cherokee tribespeople, it was taken up by European settlers and became a popular home remedy. Despite its reputation, it has been little researched to date, although it is known to contain the alkaloid berberine (see also page 91).

Harvesting
The roots are dug up from three- to four-year-old plants in autumn and dried before use. Harvest only from cultivated plants.

How to Use
Use a decoction of the roots as a gargle to alleviate sore throats, taking up to three times a day; spit once finished. For other applications, consult a qualified herbalist.

ORIGINS
Europe,
West Asia

HYPERICUM PERFORATUM

St John's wort

One of the most used herbs around the world, and one that has significant clinical evidence to support its herbal remedy uses, St John's wort has long been valued as a herb that can heal traumas, both mental and physical.

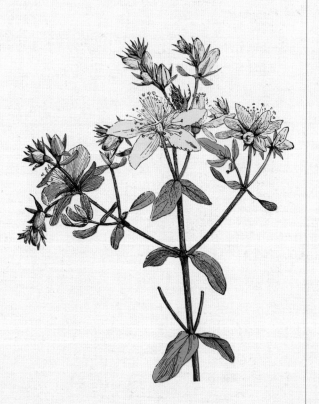

Caution
Contraindicated during pregnancy and breastfeeding and for young children. Seek professional medical advice before taking in conjunction with any prescribed medicine, including the contraceptive pill. Do not take in conjunction with prescribed antidepressants or in the case of severe depression. St John's wort can cause sensitivity to sunlight. It is restricted in some countries.

Cultivation
Considered a pervasive weed in many countries, St John's wort is difficult to eradicate once introduced to a garden. It is a hardy perennial that will grow in well-drained or dry soil in sun or shade, reaching up to 1m (3ft) tall and 60cm (2ft) wide.

A History of Healing

The earliest recorded uses of St John's wort are as a battlefield herb. Its oil was used by the Knights Hospitallers during the Crusades to heal wounds – including deep puncture wounds – where it would help to reduce inflammation and promote healing, especially of the nerve endings. It is also likely they would have needed to apply it to the soldiers for sunburn.

The 'reddish juice like blood', as described by Culpeper, that oozes from the bruised buds and flowers of St John's wort led to the plant being considered magical, but the colour is in fact due to its active constituent hypericin. Hypericin is a potent antiviral and may have potential as a treatment for HIV, chronic fatigue syndrome and other viral diseases. However, St John's wort also affects the liver, increasing the rate at which other medicines are broken down, thereby affecting their absorption and efficacy.

Although St John's wort has a long traditional use in healing nervous disorders – in France it also has the common name *chasse-diable*, or devil-chaser – it fell out of favour in the 19th century. In the late 20th century, interest in its effects as an antidepressant grew once again and it is now one of the most researched herbs in the world.

Numerous clinical trials have shown it to be useful in treating mild or moderate depression (whether or not it can successfully alleviate severe depression is still unknown), seasonal affective disorder (SAD), anxiety, low mood, especially due to menopause, and nervous exhaustion. It works on the neurotransmitters in the body, boosting serotonin levels among other things, and has fewer side-effects than prescribed antidepressants. Research has also indicated that the plant works synergistically – the whole plant has a more beneficial effect than when taken as the isolated compounds in other medicines.

Harvesting

Traditionally, the herb is harvested on the day of its eponymous saint: 24 June. Pick the flowering tops of the stems, including open flowers, buds and the top sets of leaves. Wear gloves to avoid the plant causing light sensitivity on the skin, and wash hands and arms after the harvest. Use fresh or dry, to store.

How to Use

The fresh flowers/buds can be infused in oil (which takes on a deep red colour). To harness the plant's antidepressant qualities, prepare as a tisane or tincture.

HYSSOPUS OFFICINALIS

Hyssop

Aromatic hyssop makes a striking garden plant which is extremely popular with all kinds of pollinating and beneficial insects. Hyssop extracts are used to flavour liqueurs and bitters, such as Chartreuse, and it is one of the ingredients of the Middle Eastern spice mix za'atar.

Caution
Contraindicated during pregnancy.
The essential oil should only be used
under professional supervision and can
cause epileptic seizures. It is restricted
in some countries.

Cultivation
Hyssop is a hardy perennial which will grow to 60cm (2ft) in height and spread, but it can be

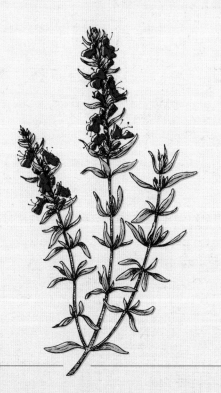

pruned back by a third in spring as well as at harvest time. It prefers well-drained or dry soil in a sunny position.

A History of Healing
Dioscorides suggested a mixture of hyssop, honey, figs and rue, and this was repeated down the ages as a remedy for all manner of bronchial complaints. Hyssop appears to thin mucus in the respiratory tract as well as being a gentle expectorant. Parkinson recommended it 'for all cold griefes or diseases of the chest and lungs, helping to expectorate tough flegme'. However, it can irritate the mucus membranes, and herbalists now prescribe it more to speed recovery than to help alleviate symptoms at their peak. Hyssop is also a general tonic for the digestion.

Harvesting
Cut whole flowering stems in summer, taking off the top third of each stem, and hang upside down to dry.

How to Use
For coughs and colds, drink as a tisane, or take as an infused honey. Young leaves and flowers were popular in many medieval dishes and can be added to food, although sparingly because they have a sage/mint flavour that can be an acquired taste for some.

ILEX PARAGUARIENSIS (SYN. I. PARAGUENSIS)

Maté *Yerba maté, Paraguay tea*

Maté is taken as a daily drink in South America, a hot-water infusion that gives a physical and mental energy boost.

Cultivation

Growing to a height of 15m (49ft) and a spread of 10m (33ft), this large evergreen tree needs a minimum temperature of 7°C (45°F), and moist, well-drained soil in full sun or shade.

A History of Healing

Similar to both tea and coffee in its properties and uses, maté is reputed to enhance short-term energy levels without the side-effects of coffee. It contains about 1.5 per cent caffeine, approximately half that of an average Americano. Maté is said to relieve pain, fatigue, depression and headaches and to clear toxins (it is a diuretic); several studies have concluded it contains high levels of antioxidants (more than green tea, see page 99). The high levels of tannins in maté inhibit nutrient absorption by the gut, so do not take maté with meals.

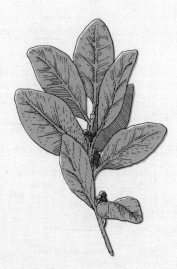

DRINKING AND BREWING MATÉ

Customarily, the drinking of maté is a communal affair, with the maté gourd being passed around after the maker (*cebador*) has had a first, testing sip. To be offered a gourd of maté is a sign of respect, and it would be rude to decline.

To make maté, you will need a maté gourd, which is the cup, and a metal straw (bombilla) with a filter at one end.

Heat the water to a maximum temperature of 85°C (185°F). Half-fill the gourd with dried and crumbled maté leaves. Put your hand over the top, then briefly invert it so the smaller, powdery pieces are on top when the gourd is righted. Tap the leaves to one side of the gourd. Add some hot water until the leaves are almost but not completely covered and leave to infuse for 5–10 minutes. Add the straw, filter end downwards, and top up with more water. The leaves can be reinfused several times over, to taste; Buenos Aires has many hot-water stations where a thermos can be refilled, ready to top up the gourd as needed.

ORIGINS
Europe,
West Asia

INULA HELENIUM

Elecampane *Scabwort, pushkaramula*

Sometimes also known as elf-dock or elf-wort, elecampane was thought in medieval times to help cure the general malaise called elf-shot, which was caused by the invisible arrows of elves. A medieval saying had it that, 'Elecampane will the spirits sustain.' This has translated into a modern use as a general tonic for chronic fatigue, but elecampane is more effective for bronchial complaints.

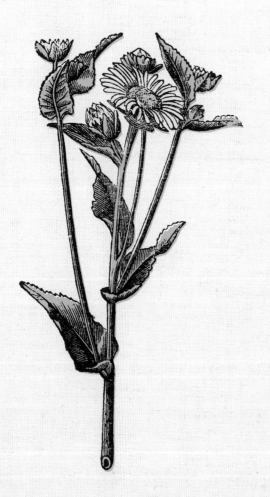

Caution
Contraindicated for pregnancy and breastfeeding. Elecampane is a member of the Asteraceae family and should be avoided by anyone with allergies to these plants.

Cultivation
A towering herbaceous perennial, elecampane resembles a multistemmed sunflower with narrow yellow petals. It can reach 2m (6½ft) or more in height, and 1.5m (5ft) in spread. Grow in moist but well-drained soil and full sun. Cut back the previous year's growth in late winter.

A History of Healing
Inulin was first discovered in the roots of elecampane, taking its name from the herb's Latin name. Elecampane roots are up to 44 per cent inulin, though modern powdered inulin is more commonly isolated from chicory roots (see page 106). A starchy substance, it has

a prebiotic effect on the gut, although it is not actually digested itself, and is also sometimes prescribed for diabetics and constipation. Pliny the Elder wrote that Julia Augustus (born 39 BCE), the daughter of the Roman emperor, 'let no day pass without eating some of the roots of Enula, considered to help digestion and cause mirth'. Elecampane roots overall are mildly bitter, and they continued to be viewed as a digestive tonic in medieval times, though generally that was secondary to their applications for bronchial complaints. Today, the roots are an ingredient in vermouth.

In Ayurvedic medicine, elecampane, known as pushkaramula, is a widely regarded tonic for the lungs and respiratory system, and it was also used in Western herbalism to shift persistent phlegm, encouraging it to be coughed up. Dr William Fernie, a Victorian doctor who wrote *Herbal Simples Approved for Modern Uses of Cure*, a guide to herbal remedies of the time, reported that 'it was customary when travelling by a river to suck a bit of the root against poisonous exhalations and bad air'. There was also a popular belief at the time in miasmas – 'bad air' that would infect and also carry disease, particularly

cholera which was prevalent at the time in the newly industrialized and crowded cities. Although science has now disproven the idea of miasmas, any tonic against the London smog and sewage-ridden river water would no doubt have been welcome. One trial has shown elecampane to be effective against the MRSA hospital superbug, so there may be further potential in this herb's constituents.

Harvesting
Dig up a portion of the roots in autumn and use fresh or dry. Flowers can be infused, but are best avoided as they contain irritant hairs – steep them within a muslin bag, if using.

How to Use
The fresh or dried roots can be decocted, or follow the advice of Parkinson and Culpeper and preserve them in a syrup instead; the roots can be chewed directly but they are more palatable when coated in sugar. The aromatic, clearing properties of the root can also be harnessed by preserving small pieces of root in a jam when they act like cough drops – nibble one at a time, and take sparingly.

ORIGINS
Europe, Asia (*J. regia*);
North America
(*J. cinerea, J. nigra*)

JUGLANS

Walnut, butternut and black walnut

The *Juglans* genus includes butternut (*J. cinerea*) – nothing to do with the pumpkin-like squash that shares its name – and black walnut (*J. nigra*), which can be used in much the same way to treat digestive complaints. Walnut (*J. regia*) has a nutritious nut, like *J. cinerea* and *J. nigra*, and its bark is used as a mild purgative as well as being applied to skin problems, but the bark does not have the same healing qualities as the other two species.

Cultivation

These large deciduous trees grow upwards of 25m (82ft) in height, depending on the species, and have wide spreading branches. They prefer a deep, rich soil in full sun and, although they are hardy, they crop better in warmer climates. Young shoots and leaves can be damaged by frost.

A History of Healing

Butternut and black walnut bark were widely used by the indigenous American people, and then European settlers, as a laxative and overall tonic for the digestion, listed in the *US Pharmacopeia* of 1820–1905 as the most widely used laxative in the country. As a remedy for constipation, it is especially effective when combined with ginger (see page 246), and it is also said to lower cholesterol levels. The husks of the nuts can be used as a dye; the Menominee tribe stained their deerskin shirts brown with them.

Harvesting

The inner bark is the part most used for its laxative effect. It is collected in autumn and dried before use.

How to Use

Drink a decoction of the bark as a laxative and purgative. Eat the nuts raw once they are ripe or pickle them when unripe.

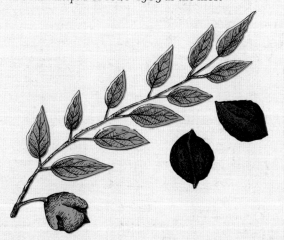

ORIGINS
North America

JUNIPERUS COMMUNIS

Juniper

The chief flavouring of gin, juniper also has culinary applications: dried berries are added to pickles and to flavour various pork and game dishes. They were held in high esteem as a herbal remedy by Culpeper in Europe as well as by Native American tribespeople.

Caution
Contraindicated during pregnancy, heavy menstrual bleeding and cases of kidney infections or kidney disease.

Cultivation
Many junipers sold as ornamental plants are male versions of the species, so be sure to source a female plant to be able to harvest the berries. An evergreen shrub, it can grow to 6m (20ft) tall and wide, but is most often seen in smaller forms. Juniper is a hardy plant and tolerates most soils and situations.

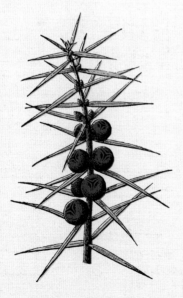

A History of Healing
Culpeper held juniper as 'scarce to be paralleled for its virtues', but he was prone to overenthusiasm. It was used as a diuretic and general tonic for the digestion and kidneys/bladder and continues to be esteemed as a herbal remedy for cystitis, being antiseptic in action, particularly so within the urinary tract. In its native America it was also used against dandruff.

Foraging and Harvesting
Ripe berries are blue-grey-black in colour, with the unripe ones green. The berries take three years to ripen, rather than growing and ripening within a summer, 'and therefore,' as Culpeper wrote, 'you shall always find upon the bush green berries'. If home-grown or foraged berries are not an option, they are widely available to buy dried in supermarkets.

How to Use
A possible irritant, juniper can be combined with demulcent herbs, such as marsh mallow (see page 80). Prepare dried berries as a decoction for the relief of cystitis. The berries can also be made into an infused oil, for a warming massage oil and moisturizer, stimulating the circulation and potentially helping to remedy cellulite, as well as bringing relief to tired muscles and period pains.

LAURUS NOBILIS

Bay laurel *Bay*

An essential component of a bouquet garni, bay has a long history in herbal medicine and plant lore.

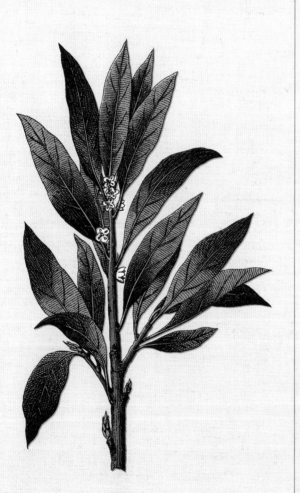

Cultivation

Evergreen bay laurel can grow to a large tree of up to 15m (49ft), but can also be kept clipped into a smaller size and shape by regular pruning. Grow in well-drained soil in full sun.

A History of Healing

Although bay is a potent antiseptic, it is more commonly used in cooking than herbal medicine today. Taken infused in food or water, it is known to assist the body breaking down heavy fats, such as those in meat, and aiding digestion in general. Culpeper warned that bay leaves 'mightily expel the wind'.

Bay laurel is also soothing to aches and pains when applied externally. It is said a poultice of the leaves draws out bee and wasp stings, and that, according to Culpeper, 'A bath of the decoction of leaves and berries, is singularly good for women to sit in.'

Harvesting

Bay leaves can be picked all year round, or whole branches can be cut and dried in summer. Use dried leaves within a year.

How to Use

Add fresh or dried bay leaves to soups and stews – they are best used for slow- or long-cooked dishes to allow them to infuse. They pair well with blackberry (see page 200) and can be infused into a jam of the fruits. An infusion of the leaves will help ease indigestion and wind, or an infused oil can be used as a massage. Leaves can be added to baths.

MYTH AND LEGEND

According to the Greek myths, the nymph Daphne was so fed up with the attentions of Apollo that she asked the gods to help her. They obliged (although perhaps not from her point of view) by turning her into a bay laurel tree, but even then she was not free of him, for he cut off some branches and wore them in a wreath around his head. Ever after the bay laurel has been known as sacred to both Apollo and to Asclepius, the gods responsible for medicine and healing.

Perhaps because of this connection with the gods, bay laurel has a number of superstitions attached to it. It is said a wreath of bay laurel on the door will keep the home both lucky and free of disease. To continue this protection while out and about, simply carry a bay leaf – in the mouth! – all day. If a bay tree dies suddenly, it is taken as an omen of imminent disaster.

Bay laurel is also indelibly associated with achievement. Victors of the early Olympic Games were garlanded with laurel wreaths – and because the Games then also included artistic competition, we take the word 'laureate' from 'laurel', as in 'poet laureate'. It is also the origin of the name of the qualification 'baccalaureate', and, derived from that through the French *bachelier*, 'bachelor's', as applied to university qualifications. Roman emperors and commoners alike were also particularly fond of bay laurel, using it as a celebratory decoration for carriages and swords, wrappings for battlefield missives, and as garlands for the December festival of Saturnalia.

ORIGINS
France, Western
Mediterranean

LAVANDULA ANGUSTIFOLIA

Lavender *English lavender*

Although known as English lavender, *L. angustifolia* actually originates in the Mediterranean. Other species include lavandin (*L.* × *intermedia*), the variety most commonly used for large-scale crops for perfume oil, and French, or butterfly, lavender (*L. stoechas*). The etymology is disputed, but one theory suggests *Lavandula* derives from the Latin *lavare*, meaning 'to wash', and certainly it has a long history of being used to scent baths, body oils, soaps and laundry. English lavender is the species best used for therapeutic purposes.

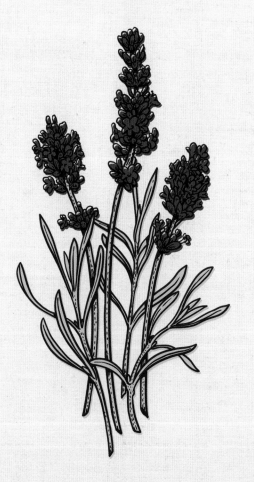

Cultivation

Native to the rocky screes and well-drained soils of the Mediterranean, lavender will produce its best flowers in poor, well-drained soils and full sun. Wetter conditions will promote lusher foliage at the expense of flowers.

To prevent the plant from sprawling and becoming too leggy – it can reach 1m (3ft) in height and spread – cut back to just above the old wood after flowering (or while harvesting) and replace plants every four years or so. Cultivars such as the more compact 'Hidcote' and 'Clarmo' (syn. 'Little Lottie') can be used interchangeably with the species.

A History of Healing

Lavender's oil has long been used for its sweet scent, initially as a perfumed oil: it has been found in the tombs of the ancient Egyptians and was widely used in the Roman Empire for bathing. The relaxing properties of the flowers and oil were more widely applied from the

Middle Ages, with several herbals noting its ability to reduce anxiety, promote sleep and generally relax the body and mind. Parkinson described it as being of 'especiall good use for all griefes and paines of the head and braine'. Lavender was one of the herbs taken by the Pilgrims to the New World in 1620, indicating its value at the time, and it was a mainstay of the English home stillroom.

The discovery of the antiseptic quality of lavender essential oil is attributed to a French chemist called René-Maurice Gattefossé in the early 20th century, when he applied lavender essential oil to burns sustained in his laboratory. Noting how fast and well the skin healed, he promoted the use of lavender oil in the army hospitals of the First World War. Lavender was one of the 'herbs of war' that the domestic population of Great Britain (including Boy Scouts and Girl Guides) was asked to collect during the Second World War, when it was used as an antiseptic and cleaning agent to supplement low stocks of medicines – the principal pharmaceutical companies in Europe were German.

Lavender's strong scent was believed to signify its magical properties: a cross made from lavender sprigs and hung on the door was said to keep the Devil from the house, and a lavender buttonhole would keep evil at bay while out and about. Folklore also suggests a sprig of lavender under a man's pillow will make him dream of the woman who put it there.

Harvesting
Harvest the flower spikes as the petals begin to fade, cutting them with a good length of stem and hanging upside down in bunches to dry. To use in dried flower arrangements, harvest as the first buds begin to open and dry in the same way.

How to Use
Lavender flowers can be used to have an all-round soothing, calming and relaxing effect and to aid a restful night's sleep: make up cotton bags of the dried flowers to put next to the bed – these can also be used as moth repellents in clothes and linen drawers – or add them to a tisane. The flowers can be used – sparingly – in cakes, biscuits and scones, and are also good with roast lamb.

Apply the essential oil neat on stings, bites and burns, and use it in massage oils and baths for a relaxing effect. Massage a few drops of essential oil into the temples to ease headaches and tension.

ORIGINS
North Africa to
Southwest Asia

LAWSONIA INERMIS (SYN. L. ALBA)

Henna *Egyptian privet, mignonette tree*

Henna is the only species in this genus, a traditional plant for windbreak hedges around vineyards. In the Bible, henna is referred to as camphire, from henna's Arabic name: 'My beloved is unto me as a cluster of camphire in the vineyards of Engedi.' Song of Solomon 1:14.

Cultivation
Henna requires a minimum temperature of 13°C (55°F), full sun and light, sandy soil. It will grow to a bushy 3–6m (10–20ft) tall and 2–4m (6½–13ft) wide, and can be kept in shape with an annual prune in late spring or early summer.

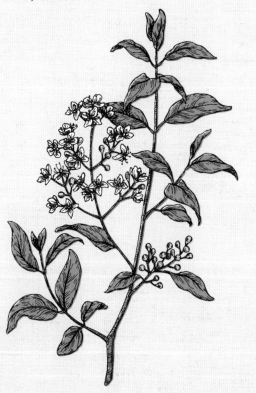

A History of Healing
It is only in Ayurvedic medicine that henna is used for any healing benefit, taken as a gargle for sore throats or a decoction for diarrhoea. Elsewhere it is its ability to impart a reddish-brown dye that has been most advantageous. The dye is used for cloth – it coloured the shrouds for mummification in Ancient Egypt, and Cleopatra allegedly dyed the sails of her barge with henna en route to meet Antony. There are records from five thousand years ago of it being combined with indigo to make a black dye. It is used also to dye the hair of people and horses as well as the intricate, delicate patterns temporarily tattooed onto the skin in India and elsewhere. Introduced into Europe in the late 19th century, henna is still used as a natural dye and hair tint today.

Harvesting
Henna dye is made from the powdered leaves that are picked as young shoots during the growing season and then dried before use.

How to Use
Henna tattoos are best applied by professionals. An infusion of the leaves can be taken as a gargle for sore throats.

ORIGINS
Europe, South and
central Russia

LEONURUS CARDIACA

Motherwort

Literally meaning mother-herb, motherwort is so named for its association with helping women through all stages of their reproductive lives, but it also has a reputation of strengthening the heart, hence the species name *cardiaca*.

Caution
Contraindicated during pregnancy.

Cultivation
A herbaceous perennial reaching 1.2m (4ft) tall and 60cm (2ft) wide, motherwort prefers well-drained but moist soil in full sun or partial shade. In the wild it prefers to grow in hedgerows.

A History of Healing
Parkinson reported motherwort to 'bee of much use for the trembling of the heart, and in faintings and swounings.' Culpeper concurred: 'There is no better herb to take melancholy vapours from the heart, to strengthen it, and make a merry, cheerful, blithe soul than this

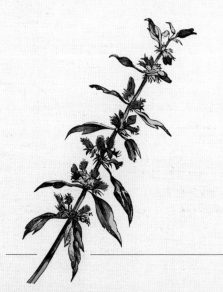

herb.' Research has proven its effectiveness in calming the heart and anxiety, and that it reduces the risk of thrombosis.

Motherwort is also associated with calming anxieties around the menopause and motherhood: 'It makes women joyful mothers of children,' wrote Culpeper, and it can promote regular periods where they are light or delayed.

Occasionally the herbal authors would recommend a herb for use in animals: Gerard says of motherwort that it is much valued by cattle-drivers and farmers as a 'remedy for certain diseases in cattell'. Juliette de Baïracli Levy (the noted 20th-century herbalist 'Juilette of the Herbs') actually started her herbal career as a herbalist for animals, rather than people, suggesting that rich grazing grounds full of herbs as well as grass would allow farm animals to self-medicate by seeking out the plants they had instinctively evolved to know would cure them.

Harvesting
Cut the flowering stems before they start to form seeds, and hang upside down in bunches to dry.

How to Use
In *A Modern Herbal*, Mrs Grieve warned that 'it has rather a pungent odour and a very bitter taste', so a tisane can be a digestive as well as a menstrual and heart tonic. Pair with other, more flavourful, herbs and/or sweeten with honey to taste.

LINUM USITATISSIMUM

Flaxseed *Linseed*

Although linseed may seem like a recent introduction to the Western diet, a new 'superfood', it has in fact been cultivated for at least seven thousand years. Its oil is used in various industrial processes and as a domestic wood treatment, such as oiling cricket bats, as well as in cooking. Waste products from oil production are used as animal feed.

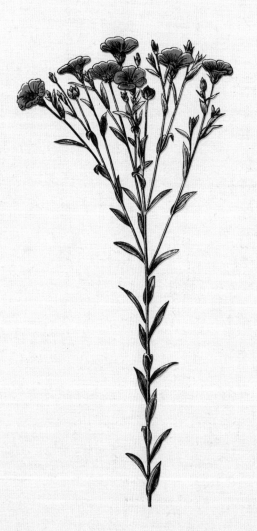

Caution
Excessive consumption can cause potentially fatal respiratory failure.

Cultivation
Well-drained or even dry soil in full sun suits flaxseed best. It will grow to around 1m (3ft) tall with a spread of 50cm (20in). This fully hardy annual can make a pretty garden plant but, as a significant area would have to be given over to them to grow enough for a decent harvest, grow the plant as a curiosity and buy the seeds from herbal suppliers.

A History of Healing
Flaxseed's benefits have still not been fully investigated, and there is ongoing research into its potential as a treatment for cancer, but it is already known that, when incorporated into the diet, flaxseed has the ability to lower the risk of prostate cancer. Flaxseed has unusually (for a plant) high levels of alpha-linolenic acid (ALA), the omega-3 'good' fat also found in oily fish and known to have an anti-inflammatory effect on the body as well as lowering cholesterol and helping cardiac health. It also contains phytoestrogenic compounds that can help balance the hormones during the menopause. Flaxseed is used for digestive health, aiding

regularity and soothing inflammation, especially in conditions such as irritable bowel syndrome, ulcerative colitis and haemorrhoids. There is also a suggestion that it is able to soothe bronchial complaints and act as an expectorant.

How to Use

Flaxseed needs to be ground or the seeds at least cracked before eating to access their oils and therapeutic compounds, but the high oil levels mean that they quickly go rancid once this has been done. The best and most economical way to use flaxseed is to buy them whole as brown or golden linseeds, then crack or grind them using a pestle and mortar or spice grinder in small batches to use straight away. Research suggests that there is no meaningful difference in the nutritional benefit of golden or brown linseeds, but the brown type taste slightly nuttier.

When taking flaxseed for the digestion, whole seeds help with easier bowel movements but ground they release their soothing mucilaginous compounds, so try a half and half mix of ground and whole seeds.

Whole seeds can be sprinkled over porridge or breakfast cereals, salads or the top of home-made breads. Ground seeds can likewise be added to many foods, especially pasta sauces, smoothies and yogurt, and the oil can be bought to use as a salad dressing. For coughs and sore throats, try infusing ground seeds in hot water and adding lemon and honey to taste.

Traditionally, flaxseeds and their flour have been mixed with other seeds to bake a 'menopause cake' or bread – they can be added to any baked goods – and they can also be used as an egg substitute in vegan cookery by mixing the ground seeds with a little water.

'MENOPAUSE MUESLI'

This muesli is rich in herbs, vitamins and minerals known to support the body through the menopause.

Mix up a large jar of the ingredients opposite, then add 2 tbsp of freshly ground flaxseed per portion before serving with milk or natural yogurt and fresh fruit. Alternatively, the night before, stir in the flaxseed and a grated apple (add a splash of milk, if liked), cover and leave in the fridge before serving with yogurt and fruit.

200g (2 cups) oats

50g (½ cup) rye flakes

50g (½ cup) buckwheat flakes

100g (¾ cup) chopped nuts (such as walnuts and almonds)

100g (¾ cup) pumpkin and/or sunflower seeds

100g (⅔ cup) raisins or sultanas

50g (¼ cup) dates, finely chopped

3 tbsp chia seeds

1 tbsp ground cinnamon (see page 108)

1 tbsp dried, powdered lady's mantle (optional, see page 72)

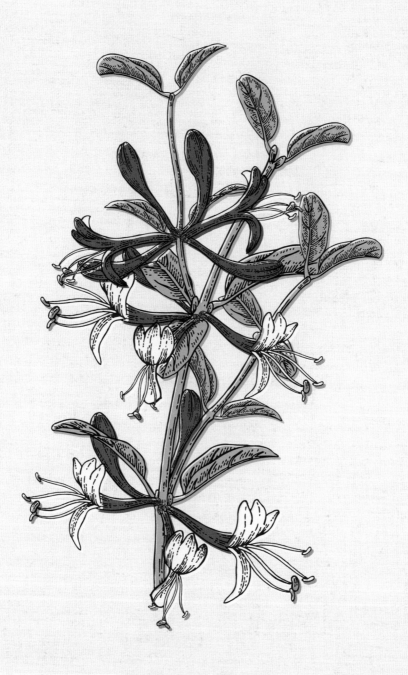

ORIGINS
East Asia

LONICERA JAPONICA

Honeysuckle *Japanese honeysuckle, Jin Yin Hua*

Lonicera japonica is the honeysuckle most used for its therapeutic properties: the other yellow-or pink-flowered species, *L. caprifolium* and *L. periclymenum*, can be substituted but are considered less effective.

Caution
The berries are considered toxic and should be avoided. Subject to legislation as an invasive species in some countries.

Cultivation
A hardy vigorous evergreen or semi-evergreen climber, honeysuckle can reach 10m (33ft) or more. Plant in well-drained soil in sun or partial shade.

A History of Healing
Honeysuckle has been important since at least *c.*659 CE when it is mentioned in the *Tang Materia Medica*. Traditional Chinese medicine views honeysuckle as a cooling herb, one that can clear excess heat and toxicity from the body in the cases of fever and the hot flushes of the menopause. The stems and flowers are used interchangeably for some complaints and separately for others. Honeysuckle is also applied to inflammatory conditions such as mastitis and conjunctivitis.

In the West, honeysuckle's cooling, soothing properties are today used mostly for bronchial complaints, such as dry coughs and sore throats. However, for a time its cooling nature was disputed. Gerard and Parkinson both argued that it was hot in nature, and should therefore not be used for inflamed conditions. Culpeper agreed with them, writing that chewing on a fresh leaf is 'likelier to cause a sore mouth and throat than to cure it', railing against 'Dr Tradition' and his power over 'Dr Reason' in the minds of the 'common people'.

As one of the flowers of the Bach Flower Remedy system, honeysuckle extracts are used for countering nostalgia and homesickness. Research has shown it to have antimicrobial properties and the ability to lower blood pressure, and to contain pain-killing salicylic acid.

Harvesting
Pick the flowers before they open in the early morning, and use fresh or dry.

How to Use
Infuse honeysuckle into honey or hot water to help relieve sore throats and (nervous) headaches and to cool hot flushes. Alternatively, make them into a cordial using the recipe on page 133, or even a jelly using the infused water or cordial.

MARANTA ARUNDINACEA

Arrowroot

Arrowroot is so called for its reputation in being able to draw out the infection from a wound caused by a poisoned arrow when applied as a poultice, but it is also a healing foodstuff.

A History of Healing
Arrowroot is most familiar as the eponymous pudding, a milky gruel often used for convalescence and weaning babies because of its high starch content and demulcent effect on the digestion, which soothes and provides some nutrition. The powder can also be used as a thickening agent in the same way as cornstarch. A staple food of the Arawak people in the Caribbean, it was introduced to Europe in the mid-18th century.

Harvesting
Arrowroot is made from the powdered rhizomes of the plant, which are dug up only 10–11 months after planting (compared with the three- to four-year-old rhizomes and roots taken from most other herbs).

How to Use
Use powdered arrowroot with milk and water to make a thin 'porridge', adding flavour with cinnamon and/or vanilla, and sugar and salt, to taste.

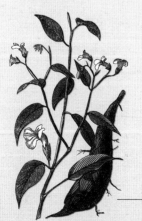

ORIGINS
Northern South America and Caribbean

MARRUBIUM VULGARE

White horehound

This has a long history in Europe, and is one of the five traditional herbs eaten at Passover, known as *marrob* (the other herbs are lettuce, nettles, coriander and horseradish). Horehound ale, a herbal beer, is made using the leaves.

Caution
Prolonged use may cause high blood pressure.

Cultivation
A hardy woody perennial that reaches around 50cm (20in) in height and spread, white horehound prefers well-drained, even poor soil in full sun. It is often found on wasteland.

A History of Healing
Dioscorides recommended a decoction of white horehound for coughs as well as more serious respiratory conditions, such as asthma and tuberculosis, and its reputation for healing bronchial complaints continues to this day. It is also a bitter herb. White horehound is today used in Mexico in cases of late onset diabetes, and has been shown to have vasodilatory properties – which supports its other traditional use of normalizing an irregular heartbeat.

How to Use
The whole plant can be infused fresh or dried into syrups to soothe a cough.

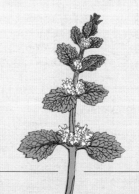

ORIGINS
Europe, Asia, North Africa

MELALEUCA ALTERNIFOLIA

Tea tree

This species has the best-quality tea tree oil, although other *Melaleuca* species are sometimes used. The constituents of the volatile oil – notably terpinen-4-ol, the main antiseptic compound in the plant – vary in percentage depending on various environmental factors. Poorer-quality oils contain higher levels of cineol, which is a skin irritant.

Cultivation
A half-hardy shrub or small tree growing up to 7m (23ft) tall and 5m (16½ft) wide, tea tree likes damp to wet soil and full sun.

A History of Healing
Traditionally used by the Aboriginal people as a remedy for skin infections, stings and wounds, tea tree's properties were first investigated in the 1920s, when the essential oil was established to be antiseptic. The oil was used as a wound dressing by the Australian army during the Second World War in much the same way lavender was by the British (see page 157).

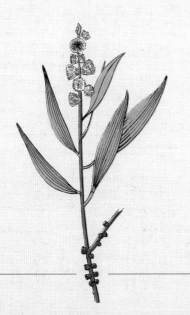

Extensive further research into the plant's properties in the 1990s proved its antiseptic qualities beyond doubt and tea tree has gained wide acceptance as a healing herb, often featuring in face washes for greasy or spot-prone skin and mouthwashes. Clinical trials have also shown the essential oil to be effective in treating a number of infections, especially those of the skin, such as warts, acne and also vaginal thrush.

The aromatic leaves can also be used to alleviate congestion, coughs and flu-like symptoms.

Harvesting
The young leaf tips are picked regularly through the year, from which the essential oil is distilled. The leaves can also be dried.

How to Use
Tea tree is best applied externally in the form of the essential oil, diluted in a carrier oil/base cream (5 drops of essential oil per tablespoon of carrier oil or base cream). Mixed in equal quantities with other essential oils such as lavender, eucalyptus and rosemary, and diluted with cider vinegar, tea tree essential oil can also be rubbed into the scalp to treat nits, but do not use on children under two and always patch-test it first. Add 3 drops of each oil to 4 tbsp of cider vinegar. Add the leaves to boiling water for steam inhalation and use for congestion.

MELISSA OFFICINALIS

Lemon balm *Balm, sweet balm, melissa*

A wonderful plant for attracting bees, lemon balm is also known as bee balm. Its popularity with pollinators was noted by Pliny the Elder and Gerard, the latter writing, 'It is profitably planted where bees are kept. The hives of bees being rubbed with bawme [balm], causeth the bees to keep together.' *Melissa* is named after a nymph of Greek mythology, a honey collector and creature at one with the bees' wisdom; *mel* is Greek for 'honey'.

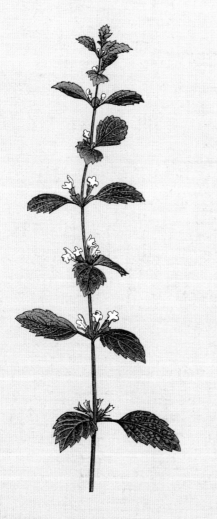

Caution
Consult a qualified herbalist before using lemon balm in the case of any thyroid condition, as there is some evidence it may inhibit thyroid function.

Cultivation
Lemon balm will grow almost anywhere and frequently does, happily seeding itself around the garden once established. It will grow bigger leaves the damper the soil, and will thrive in full sun or partial shade, provided the soil is still well drained, reaching 1m (3ft) in height and around half that in spread. Cut back after flowering, as the leaves can grow small and tatty – this will encourage fresh, lusher growth (see below). Over-large plants can be divided in spring or autumn. For pots and window boxes, grow the form 'Compacta'.

A History of Healing

Elizabeth Blackwell summed up the various properties of lemon balm thus: 'The whole Herb is used, and esteemed cordial, cephalic, good for Disorders of the Head and Nerves, chears the Heart, cures its Palpitation, prevents Fainting, Melancholy, Hypochondriac, and Hysteric Disorders.' Used since at least the 10th century CE as a remedy to ease nervous tension and lift the spirits, it was described by John Evelyn six hundred years later as 'sovereign for the brain, strengthening the memory, and powerfully chasing away melancholy'. Clinical trials have now shown that lemon balm is effective in relieving stress, anxiety, sleeplessness and poor memory by binding to receptors in the brain, indicating that it may also have potential as a treatment for sufferers of dementia.

Lemon balm is also used to soothe the digestion, especially when mental stresses or excitability are causing an irritable bowel or upset stomach, including in children. Applied externally in the form of an infused oil (the leaves yield very little essential oil), lemon balm has been shown to be effective against the herpes virus that causes cold sores.

Described by Paracelsus as the 'elixir of life', the longevity of several people was attributed by them to the lemon balm they took daily. In her herbal, Mrs Grieve tells us: 'John Hussey, of Sydenham, who lived to the age of 116, breakfasted every day on Balm tea sweetened with honey, and herb teas were the usual breakfast of Llewelyn, Prince of Glamorgan who died in his 108th year. Carmelite water, of which Balm was the chief ingredient, was drunk daily by the Emperor Charles V.'

Harvesting and Storing

Pick fresh leaves as required. The fresh leaves make a more flavourful tea than the dried, so dry only a small quantity (enough to last through the coldest months), until it comes back into growth in spring. Alternatively, chop or crush the fresh leaves into the portions of an ice-cube tray, freeze and then pop out to store in the freezer in an airtight bag or box, defrosting before use.

Cutting back the flowering stems (after the bees have had their fill) encourages fresh growth – these stems can be added to the bath for a floral soak.

How to Use

Lemon balm is best infused in hot water and drunk as an all-round calming tea, but the fresh leaves can also be infused in cold water, or made into a cordial (see page 133 for a recipe). Add the leaves (and flowers) to salads or substitute in part for other herbs in home-made pesto. Stir lemon balm-infused honey into hot water or drizzle it over a breakfast porridge ahead of a busy or worrying day (such as exams for schoolchildren).

Add flowering stems to the bath (see above), and use an infused oil as a moisturizer or massage oil, or as an ingredient for creams and salves.

ORIGINS
West and central
Europe

MENTHA X PIPERITA

Peppermint *Mint*

Peppermint tea is one of the most widely known tisanes in the West, and often one of only two choices of herbal tea on a menu. Incredibly easy to grow, and mild enough to use regularly, it is a valuable addition as a garden plant as well as a home remedy.

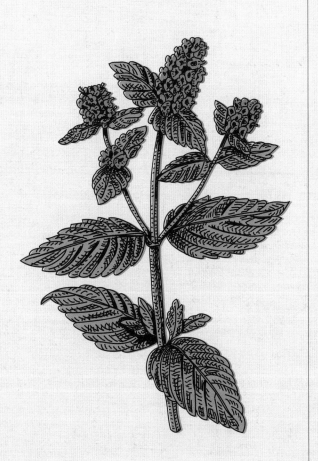

Peppermint is actually a hybrid plant of water mint (*M. aquatica*) and spearmint (*M. spicata*), which originate from Europe and Western Asia.

Caution
Although mint is helpful for the digestion, it should not be used in cases of heartburn, acid reflux or hiatus hernia, as there is some evidence that it can exacerbate these conditions.

Cultivation
Mint likes damp but well-drained, rich soil, in full sun or partial shade. It is a hardy herbaceous perennial that reaches around 50cm (20in) in height but roots and spreads widely and readily, and so can be best grown in a pot to prevent it from being invasive. As Parkinson wrote, mint roots are 'so plentifull, that being once planted in a garden, they are hardly rid out againe, every small piece thereof being left in the ground increasing far enough.' The middle of the plant eventually dies out as it spreads, which is particularly obvious in pot-grown mints.

To keep it fresh, divide the plant and replant just a quarter of it back into the pot in new compost. For fresh leaves in winter, cut off a piece of stolon (the whitish roots that grow over the top of the ground) and put it in a glass of water on the windowsill. It should soon root and shoot, and can be potted up to keep indoors.

A History of Healing

Remains of mint leaves have been found in the tombs of the Ancient Egyptians. It was a popular remedy for the Ancient Greeks and Romans, with Dioscorides writing that it was a hot herb, though it is generally now considered cooling. Mint's name is said to derive from Menthe, another unfortunate Greek nymph who was turned into a plant (see also page 155), this time by Persephone who was jealous of the love between Menthe and Pluto.

Western herbalism largely used, and uses, mint as a herb to aid the digestion, where it is soothing and carminative. Capsules of the oil are given as an over-the-counter medicine for irritable bowel syndrome, but research has also shown the efficacy of the whole herb. Culpeper summarized it thus: 'Briefly, it is very profitable to the stomach'.

Menthol, a constituent of mint's volatile oil, is a well-known decongestant, and mint taken as a tea or strewn in a bath, or used for steaming, can help to clear catarrh; it is also used as an aromatic flavouring in various products, including toothpaste. Mint's association with fresh breath dates back millennia, with the leaves most commonly simply chewed to sweeten the mouth, but Mrs Grieve wrote in *A Modern Herbal* that it was also used to whiten the teeth in the 14th century.

The menthol in peppermint essential oil can be an irritant, but once diluted and dabbed onto the temples it can bring relief from a headache.

Harvesting

Pick mint regularly to use fresh through the growing season. Cut whole stems to dry, using the dried herb within a year.

How to Use

Infuse fresh or dried mint in hot water for a relaxing tea that will aid digestion and reduce bloating. Fresh mint can also be infused in cold water – it's especially good with added lemon – or made into a refreshing mint and ginger cordial. Add the fresh leaves and flowers to salads, or use in cooking, for example, chopped with fresh parsley (see page 183) and sprinkled over the top of dishes, or made into mint sauce.

OTHER MINT SPECIES AND CULTIVARS

Mint species are often variable and prone to hybridizing with each other, so the exact number of species in the genus is disputed. Some other mints worth growing include:

Black peppermint (*M.* x *piperita* 'Black Peppermint') is an attractive black-stemmed version of peppermint, with a hint of spice to the leaves.

Apple mint (*M. suaveolens*) can be used to infuse drinks, but its tall stems of glaucuous, furry leaves are also a great filler for cut-flower arrangements.

Strawberry mint (*M.* x *piperita* 'Strawberry') has a fragrance, a delicious mix of strawberries and mint, just as its name suggests. For this reason it is ideal for garnishing or infusing into fruit-based desserts and drinks, and is excellent in a Pimm's.

Chocolate mint (*M.* x *piperita* f. *citrata* 'Chocolate') is another fragranced mint, and adds a tasty dimension to a mint tea.

Spearmint (*M. spicata*), also known as garden mint, is the mint of mint sauce. It is also the better choice for cold drinks and cocktails, such as mojitos, but the best mint for a mint julep is the variety 'Kentucky Colonel'.

Moroccan mint (*M. spicata* var. *crispa* 'Moroccan'), makes a delicious mint tea – but there are several different versions under this cultivar name available from different plant nurseries. Find the one you like best – the version sold by plant hunter Paul Barney of Edulis nursery was collected by him from Morocco and is highly recommended.

MYRRHIS ODORATA

Sweet cicely

Sweet cicely is the only species in this genus. It is quick into growth in spring, and is often paired with its early spring partner rhubarb, both to reduce the amount of sugar needed and add a gentle aniseed flavour. The seeds also have culinary uses, both savoury and sweet.

Cultivation
Sweet cicely grows best in moist, rich soil in full sun or shade. It is a herbaceous perennial and fully hardy. It will reach 1–2m (3–6½ft) tall with a spread of 60cm–1.2m (2–4ft).

A History of Healing
Generally, sweet cicely is used as a culinary or salad herb rather than a medicinal one but Culpeper wrote that 'the candied roots…are held as effectual as Angelica, to preserve from infection in the time of a plague, and to warm and comfort a cold weak stomach.'

Tips for Growing
The leaves, roots and seeds can all be used. To harvest the seeds and a fresh supply of leaves through the season, grow at least two plants, cutting one back after flowering to stimulate fresh leaf growth and allowing the other to seed.

How to Use
Infuse the leaves in hot water, cook with fruit or add fresh to salads. Cook the roots as a vegetable or eat cooked and cold in salads. All parts of the plant can help ease digestion and coughs and colds.

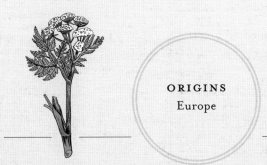

ORIGINS
Europe

MYRTUS COMMUNIS

Myrtle

Myrtle is associated with the Greek goddess of love Aphrodite, and to this day it is traditional for brides to carry a sprig of myrtle in their wedding bouquet.

Cultivation
Myrtle is only borderline hardy, suffering in severe cold and/or wet winters. An evergreen shrub, it will reach up to 3m (10ft) in height and spread, and prefers well-drained soil in full sun.

A History of Healing
Dioscorides wrote that myrtle was a 'friend to the stomach', and the leaves have an antiseptic quality thought to help heal digestive and urinary problems. The leaves are also astringent, and have been used to treat wounds. The oil is used to treat infections of the lungs and respiratory tract in Spain.

Harvesting
Pick leaves to use fresh as needed throughout the year, but don't pick too heavily in winter.

How to Use
Use the leaves to infuse savoury dishes such as stews – they have the aroma of juniper and bay, and the dried berries can be used in place of juniper berries for cooking. Infuse the leaves in hot water as a tonic drink, or add to a steam inhalation bowl for colds and congestion.

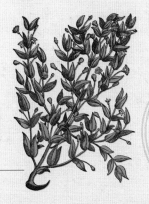

ORIGINS
Mediterranean and Southwest Europe

OCIMUM TENUIFLORUM (SYN. *O. SANCTUM*)

Holy basil *Tulsi*

Primarily an Ayurvedic herb, holy basil is closely related to sweet basil, *O. basilicum*, the culinary species most commonly used to garnish pizzas and make pesto sauce. All basils are strongly aromatic; *O. campechianum*, which is grown in the Caribbean, is used as a mosquito repellent, but all basils have some insect-repelling qualities. They are therefore useful grown on windowsills or around doorways, and also around fruit and vegetable plots, to discourage flies and pests from the house and garden.

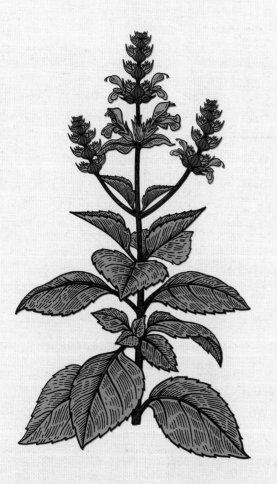

Caution
Contraindicated during pregnancy or if trying to conceive (including for men).

Cultivation
Sow basil under cover in spring – as it is a tender perennial, it will need protection from a greenhouse, polytunnel or windowsill for most of the year, but can be moved outside in the height of summer when temperatures do not drop below 10°C (50°F). Cooler temperatures can cause the leaves to become thicker and less aromatic, so it may be best kept indoors all year round. It will need full sun and light, well-drained soil. Holy basil can reach up to 60cm (2ft) tall and 30cm (12in) wide.

A History of Healing

Second only to the lotus in the Ayurvedic order of sacred plants, holy basil is associated with the Hindu goddess Lakshmi, wife of the god Vishnu, preserver of life. It is regarded as an overall invigorating tonic – the Hindi name *tulsi* means 'matchless' – acting as an adaptogen and improving vitality and longevity. Most Hindu homes and temples have holy basil growing around them; for protection while on the move, a necklace made from dried holy basil stems can be worn.

Ayurvedic medicine uses holy basil mainly to treat fever and infection, often combining it with ginger (see page 246), black pepper (see page 186) and honey, and research has supported this application. Holy basil is known to be anti-inflammatory and analgesic, and to inhibit sperm production. Research is ongoing into its usefulness during cancer treatment, as it may be able to protect against radiation and strengthen the immune system. Generally the leaves are the most used, but the seeds have similar properties and can be taken for cold and flu relief.

Harvesting

Growing more than one plant allows for plenty of fresh leaves and also seed harvests. Pick the leaves all through the year, to encourage the plant to branch and become bushy. To dry the leaves, cut the whole plant just before flowering and hang upside down. Harvest the seeds when they are ripe and dry, to use in decoctions.

How to Use

Infuse fresh or dry leaves in hot water for a spiced tonic drink, adding ginger and honey in the case of a cold, with optional crushed black peppercorns. The leaves can be infused into honey and taken in the case of sore throats, coughs and colds. The leaves can also be used in cooking, especially in Thai dishes. Decoct or soak the seeds for at least 5 minutes before taking; longer soaking will make them more gelatinous. Simply inhaling the plant's delicious aroma (which in itself encourages some calming deep breaths) direct from the plant or through steam inhalation can help relieve headaches and feelings of stress.

OENOTHERA BIENNIS

Evening primrose

Evening primrose is not related to primroses (see *Primula*, page 190) at all, and is so called because its yellow flowers open only at night. In the language of flowers, evening primrose was assigned the meaning 'silent love', as described by the 19th-century Romantic poet John Clare (1793–1864) in these lines from his poem *Evening Primrose*:

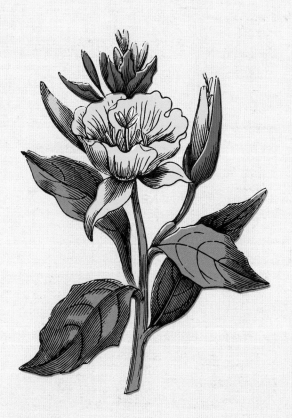

'Almost as pale as the moonbeams are,
Or its companionable star,
The Evening Primrose opens anew
Its delicate blossom to the dew;
And hermit-like, shunning the light,
Wastes its fair blooms upon the night,
Who, blindfold to its fair caresses,
Knows not the beauty it possesses.'

Caution

Contraindicated for sufferers of epilepsy and schizophrenia. Excess can cause abdominal pain and a laxative effect.

Cultivation

Sow seeds in autumn, transplanting the seedlings to their flowering position the following spring. Evening primrose will grow up to 1.5m (5ft) tall but only 25cm (10in) wide. It prefers full sun and will grow on most soils.

A History of Healing

The flowers, leaves and 'bark' of the plant were traditionally used for digestive and bronchial complaints – in her book *A Modern Herbal*, Mrs Grieve reported its use for whooping cough – and also 'in certain female complaints, such as pelvic fullness', although it is not clear here if Mrs Grieve meant an infusion of the aerial parts of the plant or the extracted seed oil.

The seed oil is now the chief use of the plant. Known to be high in gamma-linolenic acid (GLA) and other essential fatty acids, the oil has been the subject of many trials and much research, as scientists and doctors attempt to establish whether or not it can have a beneficial effect on conditions as disparate as eczema, high blood pressure, multiple sclerosis, menopausal symptoms and PMS, dementia, pancreatic cancer and heart disease. To date, some studies show positive effects but others show no discernible difference, and more research is needed.

Harvesting

Leaves and flowers can be picked and used fresh. At the end of the summer, pick the remaining leaves and flowers and peel off the top surface of the stem (the 'bark') – all these can be dried.

The primary commercial use of evening primrose is for its oil, which is pressed from the seeds and combined with vitamin E oil to prevent oxidization. A home garden harvest will not supply sufficient seeds to create a significant volume of oil, so while it could be attempted as an interesting experiment, it is best to buy good-quality oil from herbal suppliers.

How to Use

The oil can be taken in capsules, where it may help to level out the hormonal swings associated with the menstrual cycle and menopause, and may have a positive effect on skin conditions, skin elasticity and aging joints. Always follow the packet directions for dosage amounts. The oil can also be applied externally to moisturize dry and problem skin. A hot-water infusion of the flowers and/or leaves and bark may help alleviate coughs.

ORIGANUM VULGARE | ORIGANUM MARJORANA

Oregano and marjoram

Origanum derives from the Greek for 'bitter herb', and this generalized name indicates some of the confusion over the identification of oregano and marjoram. Their similar growth habits both vary depending on their situation, so the species cannot reliably be determined by size. In general, oregano (*O. vulgare*) has pink/purple flowers and marjoram (*O. marjorana*) pale pink/white flowers, but again this can vary. Furthermore, they hybridize freely with each other, creating seedlings with genes of both species. To be sure of your plants, buy from a trusted source and keep them labelled in the garden!

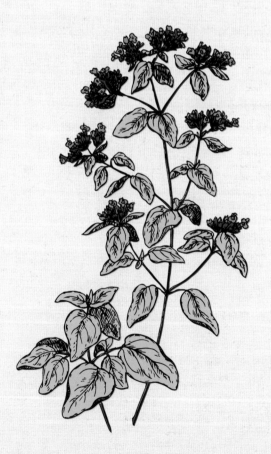

Caution
Contraindicated during pregnancy. External use of the oil may cause skin irritation.

Cultivation
Grow both species in well-drained soil and full sun. They will reach around 60–75cm (2–2½ft) tall and 40cm (16in) wide. Cut back any unharvested flower stems after flowering to keep growth bushy and trim.

A History of Healing
Marjoram and oregano have long histories of use in Western herbalism. Both were popular medieval and Tudor herbs – oregano was one of the herbs taken by settlers to the New World, and marjoram was used both medicinally and for perfume – and were strewn on the floor and 'in all odiferous waters, powders &c. that are for ornament and delight', according to Parkinson.

Oregano is known more today as a culinary herb, but the bitter qualities of the leaves stimulate the digestion, while the antimicrobial qualities of the oil make it effective against gastric infections and bacteria, such as *E. coli*. It is known to inhibit the gut flora, and can be useful when harmful gut bacteria cause bloating and wind (gut dysbiosis).

The antiseptic and antimicrobial action of oregano's oil (due to a compound called thymol) also makes it useful in the treatment of toothache and respiratory infections, including tonsillitis, and the plant's overall antioxidant effect has led to research into its potential as a treatment for cancer and liver disease.

Marjoram can be used for digestive complaints in the same way as oregano. It is thought to have a more potent effect than oregano on the nervous system, and herbalists use it as a general tonic for anxiety, insomnia and headaches caused by stress. It is also gently warming and stimulative, and can be used in the case of colds and flu. Gerard recommended it thus: 'Sweet marjoram is a remedy against cold diseases of the braine and head, being taken away to your best liking; put up into the nostrils it provokes sneesing, and draweth forth much baggage flegme [phlegm].'

Valued in classical times as 'marvellous in virtue and useful for many purposes', according to the Ancient Greek philosopher and botanist Theophrastus, the related species *O. dictamnus*, or 'dittany of Crete', was used as a wound healer and poison antidote as well as general cure-all, although its fussiness in cultivation has led to its decline in use outside Mediterranean countries.

Harvesting
Pick fresh leaves as needed. To dry, cut (flowering) stems and hang upside down.

How to Use
Oregano and marjoram leaves and flowers can be widely used fresh or dry in cooking (dried marjoram is a principal ingredient in za'atar as well as *herbes de Provence* mixes). For coughs and colds and to ease anxiety, infuse marjoram leaves in hot water, leaving for up to four hours to increase the strength. Add honey to taste.

Add oregano leaves to steam inhalation bowls to ease congestion, or infuse in hot water and drink as a digestive aid. The diluted essential oil can be used as a massage rub to relax and warm, but patch-test first.

ORIGINS
Korea and
Northeast China

PANAX GINSENG

Ginseng *Ren Shen*

Ginseng is perhaps one of the most famous herbs of traditional Chinese medicine, and has been used for over five thousand years as a tonic. So prized was this herb that wars were fought over control of the forests in which it grew best. It is now extremely rare in the wild, and its cultivation requires a good degree of horticultural skill.

Caution
Excessive consumption can cause side-effects, including high blood pressure; do not exceed the dose or take for more than six consecutive weeks. Do not take with caffeine. Contraindicated for pregnancy, depression and anxiety, and acute inflammatory diseases.

Cultivation
Ginseng is grown from ripe seed in spring; germination is generally patchy and slow. Once established, it is hardy, and requires rich, moist but well-drained soil in shade and high humidity and heat during the growing season. A perennial, it is grown for four to seven years before the roots are lifted in autumn and dried.

A History of Healing
Ginseng is used in TCM both in combination with other herbs and on its own. It is used as a qi tonic – a vital essence – largely by people in late middle age and the elderly, and as an adaptogenic herb for athletes and those subjected to a period of stress such as exams. It is also thought to be an aphrodisiac.

Ginseng did not initially catch on in Western medicine, despite several (re-)introductions from the 9th century onwards. However, once it was established as an adaptogen in the 1950s, research has been extensive and detailed. It has been proven to improve immune function and help the body manage periods of extreme mental and physical stress (including cancer treatment); maintain virility and vitality in aging men and help alleviate symptoms of the menopause, including hot flushes and low libido.

Tips for Buying
Red and white ginseng are both dried root and originate from the same plant, but are processed in different ways. Ginseng is usually only available to buy dried. Siberian ginseng is a different species (*Eleutherococcus*).

How to Use
Dried root can be added to vegetable soups and broths (1g/¼ teaspoon per portion). Various proprietary ginseng teas are available, or prepare a tisane or tincture of the dried root.

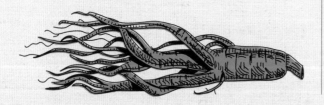

ORIGINS
Southern USA,
Central and South
America

PASSIFLORA INCARNATA

Passionflower *Passiflora, maypop, apricot vine*

Passionflower was named by European missionaries for the flower's various parts that correspond to the story of Christ's Passion (five petals for each wound, three stigma for the nails and the radial filaments for the crown of thorns) rather than any influence on the libido. Its primary use has rather the opposite effect – it is widely used as a sedative.

Cultivation
Passionflower prefers well-drained, sandy soil in full sun. A perennial climber, it is hardy, and will reach 2–8m (6½–26ft) tall each year; cut back the stems in early spring.

A History of Healing
Passionflower is widely used in the herbal traditions of Central and North America for its sedative properties, which have now been proven in clinical trials. One trial found passionflower to be as effective as the synthetic tranquillizer oxazepam, with fewer of the associated side-effects, while another found passionflower combined with hops and valerian improved sleep quality. Passionflower tablets are available as an over-the-counter remedy for stress and insomnia. Herbalists also use it as a pain remedy, particularly for period pain and headaches, and to alleviate symptoms of Parkinson's disease.

Harvesting
Flowers and leaves can be picked in summer to use fresh or to dry. Plants may produce fruit (passionfruit) in a good year, but the species *P. edulis* is normally chosen for its fruiting ability.

How to Use
When suffering from short-term or occasional insomnia, try an infusion of passionflowers and/or the leaves in hot water to make a relaxing, calming tea before bed, adding lemon balm for flavour and its own comforting properties (see page 166). Alternatively, combine in a tisane with valerian, hops and/or chamomile. Passionflower can also be prepared as a tincture and taken to help calm a busy mind.

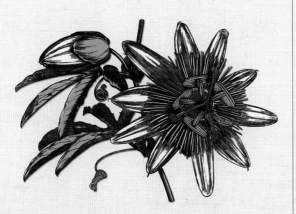

ORIGINS
Brazil, Uruguay,
Venezuela

PAULLINIA CUPANA VAR. *SORBILIS* (SYN. *P. SORBILIS*)

Guaraná *Brazilian cocoa, zoom*

Guaraná's alternative common name, zoom, gives a clue to its stimulant properties and main use as a coffee alternative. The usual species given as the source of guaraná, *P. cupana*, is now rare in the wild; *P. cupana* var. *sorbilis* is the preferred species for the widespread cultivation of the crop in South America.

Caution
Contraindicated during pregnancy and breastfeeding; and for cardiovascular disease or high blood pressure.

Cultivation
Guaraná is an evergreen vine climbing to 10m (33ft). It needs a minimum temperature of 18°C (64°F) and moist, rich soil in partial shade.

A History of Healing
Guaraná is to the Brazilian Amazon tribespeople as important as tea and coffee are to the rest of the world. Possessing properties similar to coffee, it is also drunk in hot water, though the ground seeds do not dissolve in the same way, leaving a

(nutritious) sediment in the cup and fatty film on the drink's surface. It was first brought to the attention of the rest of the world by a Jesuit missionary in 1669, but commercial plantations were not established until the 1970s.

Known to contain around 7 per cent caffeine, guaraná is used as a short-term stimulant to overcome fatigue and relieve headaches, and also for its astringent properties to treat diarrhoea. However, it contains high levels of tannins, which impair the digestion in the long-term, and, as with coffee, excessive and/or long term use can inhibit the body's ability to repair itself.

How to Use
Guaraná can be bought as a powder from herbal suppliers and prepared as a hot drink.

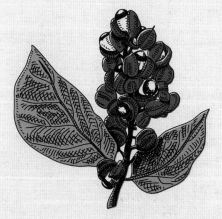

GUARANÁ PRODUCTION

The hand-pressing technique produces a superior product to the machine-made version, which allows the seeds to oxidize, making the final drink more bitter, which causes irritation of the intestines. Traditionally, the seeds are dried and powdered, then mixed with water to make a dough. The dough is rolled into sticks and dried. To use, the sticks are grated into hot water.

PELARGONIUM SIDOIDES

African geranium

Since 1724 the glasshouses at the Chelsea Physic Garden have shown a number of different species of scented pelargoniums, demonstrating their beauty and scent – they make delightful house plants. In the 21st century, scientists have used the collection to research their evolutionary relationships and DNA sequencing.

P. sidoides is very similar to *P. reniforme*, and the two species are often used interchangeably.

Cultivation
Pelargoniums are frost tender, but can be grown as house plants that are moved outside for summer. Keep them to size by cutting back to a framework in spring and autumn. Grow in well-drained soil in full sun.

A History of Healing
'Umckaloabo' is a Zulu and Xhosa word, which, in South Africa, is applied to cold and flu remedies derived from the plant, including as a brand name. Pelargonium roots have been used for centuries by South African traditional healers to treat coughs, bronchial infections and digestive upsets. The roots reputedly came to Western attention when a young Englishman called Charles Stevens arrived in South Africa with tuberculosis (TB) – at the time an incurable disease – yet he was healed when a local witch doctor gave him pelargonium root. Returning to the UK, he tried to market the herb as Stevens' Consumption Cure in the early 1900s. He met with success initially but the British Medical Association (BMA) sought to discredit him. Stevens sued the BMA for libel but lost, and was ruined.

Stevens' cure caught the attention of a Swiss doctor in the 1930s, leading to the continued use of umckaloabo as a cold and flu remedy in Germany and Russia, and it has been the recent subject of UK research into TB treatments. Although TB is now treatable, incidences are on the increase and new strains are proving resistant to the usual synthetic drug treatments, so alternatives are being sought in the natural world. Research suggests that umckaloabo appears to enhance the activity of phagocytes, the white blood cells responsible for engulfing and removing germs from the body.

Harvesting
Unearth the roots in autumn and dry before use.

How to Use
A tincture of the roots can be taken as a general immunity-boosting tonic and to help reduce the symptoms and duration of colds, flu and other respiratory infections.

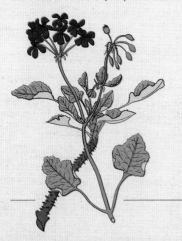

PERSEA AMERICANA

Avocado *Alligator pear*

Avocado is, of course, a nutritious and protein-rich fruit (and reputed aphrodisiac), but the fruit, leaves and bark all have herbal applications as well.

Caution
Leaves and bark are contraindicated during pregnancy.

Cultivation
Avocado trees can grow 10–15m (33–49ft) in height and spread, and require well-drained soil in full sun, high humidity and a minimum temperature of 10°C (50°F), but ideally in the 20–28°C (68–82°F) range. Fruiting is unlikely in potted glasshouse specimens in temperate climates; the dwarf variety 'Little Cado' is more suited to container growing.

A History of Healing
Traditional uses of avocado include applying the seed oil to the scalp to stimulate hair growth, and eating the fruit rind to eliminate the body of worms. The leaves and bark are typically used as a remedy for diarrhoea, and can also stimulate menstruation and induce abortion.

Modern research has shown that extracts from the leaf inhibit the herpes simplex virus (the strain responsible for cold sores and genital herpes) and that the fruit can help to lower cholesterol levels.

Harvesting
Leaves and bark can be harvested fresh as needed, or used dried. The various species of the avocado fruit differ in the rind thickness and peeling ability, but all contain similar levels of nutrients.

How to Use
Incorporate the fruit into the diet. The leaves and bark can be decocted to take in small quantities to help relieve diarrhoea. Seed oil (available from herbal suppliers) can be massaged into the skin as a moisturizer, especially for dry skin conditions, and into the scalp to aid hair growth.

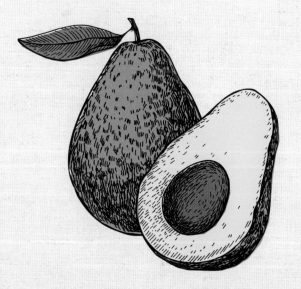

PETROSELINUM CRISPUM

Parsley

Flat- and curly-leaved parsley vary in their strength of flavour and texture on the palate, but can be viewed as much the same therapeutically. Hamburg parsley, the variant cultivated for its edible root, has inferior leaves.

Caution
Avoid in large quantities during pregnancy. Toxic in excess. Take the seeds only under professional supervision and avoid in cases of kidney disease.

Cultivation
Hasten the seeds' long germination time by soaking them overnight in water before sowing. A hardy biennial, parsley has a long taproot that needs space to grow if the plant is to thrive – allow it a large pot or plant in the ground, in rich soil and full sun or partial shade. It will reach around 30cm (12in) in height and spread.

A History of Healing
Parsley was a popular herb in Ancient Rome as an overall digestive aid and diuretic. Culpeper wrote that parsley is 'very comfortable to the stomach; helps to provoke urine.' His more questionable application was to put the leaves fried in butter on the skin, which 'takes away black and blue marks coming of bruises or falls.'

Parsley is now known to be extremely nutritionally rich, full of iron, antioxidant flavonoids and vitamins (especially A, C and K). As a diuretic, it is used by herbalists to flush out waste products from the body, with the aim of reducing the inflammation associated with gout, rheumatism and arthritis.

How to Use
Parsley leaves can be harvested fresh as needed. Their nutritional content decreases on cooking, so add to hot dishes just before serving.

Parsley leaves can be used finely chopped to make gremolata, sauces for meat and fish, or substituted for basil in home-made pesto sauce (use walnuts instead of pine nuts, too). They are also a staple ingredient of tabbouleh and excellent in salads and with new potatoes. A couple of leaves of parsley chewed on their own can help negate garlic and onion breath. The leaves can also be infused in hot water, especially in the case of urinary infections, but are more palatable eaten raw.

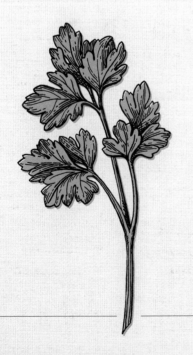

PIMENTA DIOICA

Allspice *Jamaica pepper, pimento*

Not to be confused with mixed spice (proprietary combinations of culinary spices such as cinnamon, nutmeg and coriander), allspice is a single plant but so named by the 17th-century botanist John Ray because the berries have hints of nutmeg, cinnamon and cloves.

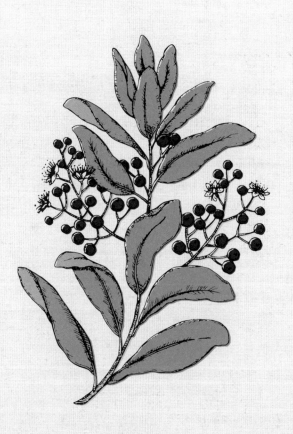

Cultivation
The evergreen allspice tree needs a minimum temperature of 15°C (59°F), rich sandy soil and full sun. It can reach a height and spread of 5m (16½ft).

A History of Healing
Allspice berries are rich in volatile oils, notably eugenol, which is also found in cloves (see page 222). They are used as a digestive tonic and stimulant, while the antiseptic and analgesic oil is applied externally for aches and pains. In Costa Rica, allspice is a traditional menopause remedy; recent research found that the berries stimulate the body's production of oestrogen and may well assist in the relief of menopausal symptoms.

Tips for Buying
Allspice berries are sold dried and whole or dried and ground, but are best bought whole and ground freshly as needed.

How to Use
Add allspice to culinary dishes – it is widely used in chutneys and pickling, as well as sauces, condiments and baking, and is an essential ingredient in Jamaican jerk seasoning mixes.

PIMPINELLA ANISUM

Anise *Aniseed*

Familiar to many from aniseed balls, the traditional sweet-shop treat, anise seeds are also the flavouring for liqueurs such as ouzo and pastis.

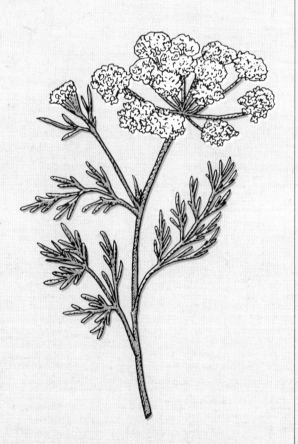

Caution
Consume only in small quantities used in cooking during pregnancy.

Cultivation
An annual reaching 50cm (20in) tall and half as much wide, anise is half-hardy and needs well-drained soil in sun. It is recommended as a companion plant for the vegetable patch, and may deter pests as well as attracting beneficial insect predators. The seed only ripens in long, hot summers.

A History of Healing
Anise has largely been a culinary flavouring, but it was also used to treat digestive disorders and coughs. Further traditional uses to encourage both the libido and lactation in nursing mothers is supported by modern research, which has established its volatile oil contains 70–90 per cent anethole, which is known to have an oestrogenic effect.

Harvesting
Be certain of correct identification when gathering seeds from the garden or the wild, as many other plants with similar flowers and seedheads are poisonous.

How to Use
Anise seeds can be taken lightly crushed and infused in hot water or added to cooking. They are still used as an ingredient in some natural cough drops.

PIPER

Black pepper, kava kava and matico

Kava, Hu Jiao (black peppercorns)

The *Piper* genus of plants includes the black pepper used as a seasoning (*P. nigrum*), the popular Polynesian drink kava from the *P. methysticum* vine, and *P. angustifolium*, or matico, from South America.

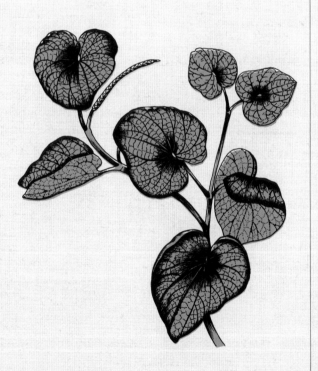

Caution
Kava should not be taken during pregnancy or breastfeeding, never to excess, not for more than two consecutive months and only in the form of water-based extracts. Kava is illegal or restricted in some countries.

Cultivation
The whole *Piper* genus requires a minimum temperature of 15°C (59°F) and high humidity – mimicking, in other words, their tropical habitat. Black pepper vines can be attempted as a house plant or greenhouse crop in a temperate climate, given rich, well-drained soil and light shade. Cut back the vines to 30cm (12in) several times a year to stimulate new growth, keeping and tying in only the ten strongest shoots, which will grow to around 4m (13ft).

A History of Healing
Black pepper is one of the oldest-known, and most widely traded, spices in the world. It was the primary spice carried along the ancient caravan trading routes from East to West, and still accounts for a quarter of the world spice market today. Pepper was once so valuable that Attila the Hun demanded it as a ransom as he lay siege to Rome, and landlords would rent out their properties for it (a peppercorn rent).

The wealth and status of Venice was built upon the sea trading routes that the city's merchants sought out primarily to better compete in the trade of pepper.

The Western, Ayurvedic and traditional Chinese medicine traditions all view black pepper as warming, to be used internally for digestive stimulus and as an expectorant in the case of congestion. It is known that pepper's chief active constituent, piperine, is anti-inflammatory and an antioxidant and has potential anticancer properties. Piperine is also known to assist the body in absorbing other herbs, notably turmeric (see page 118).

Kava kava is indigenous to the Polynesian islands, where it is extremely culturally significant, playing a large role in day-to-day life as well as ritual ceremonies. It is unusual among *Piper* crops in that it is the root that is used, not the fruit or leaves; traditionally the dried root is chewed and fermented with saliva before being made into a drink. In small doses it calms the mind and makes it more alert; larger doses lead to intoxication and euphoria and a numbing of the mouth. It is regarded as an aphrodisiac and also a remedy for anxiety and chronic pain. Kava kava is also used as a urinary antiseptic in the treatment of cystitis and other urinary tract infections.

Matico is also a urinary antiseptic, though it is the leaves of this shrub that are used, gathered fresh from the wild or cultivated plants through the year. It is also traditionally used for a wide range of gastrointestinal problems, including internal bleeding and haemorrhoids.

Tips for Buying

Black, white and green peppercorns differ only in their processing – all will contain piperine and other beneficial compounds. Black and green peppercorns are picked unripe and dried, or unripe and pickled (green only); white peppercorns are picked ripe and retted, or soaked, before drying.

Kava and, to a lesser extent, matico are available to buy as dried roots and leaves or proprietary tea blends.

How to Use

Use black pepper in infused oils and decoctions, or grind into infusions such as golden milk (see page 119) and food. Limit kava tea consumption to one or two cups per day. Dried matico leaves can be prepared as a tisane.

ORIGINS
Europe,
temperate Asia

PLANTAGO

Plantain and psyllium

The plantain species found in UK gardens, meadows and hedgerows (*P. major* and the narrower-leaved *P. lanceolata*) are so common and easily spread that they are considered a weed by most. As European settlers spread across North America, plantains became known among the indigenous people as 'white man's foot', from their habit of springing into growth in their path. The 19th-century American poet Henry Longfellow refers to this in *The Song of Hiawatha*:

> 'Wheresoe'er they tread, beneath them
> Springs a flower unknown among us,
> Springs the White-man's Foot in blossom'

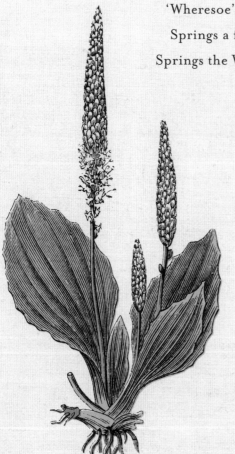

Psyllium is the seed product, also known as flea seed (referring to their small, black appearance) and *ispaghula* in Hindi, which derives mainly from *P. psyllium*, *P. ovata* and *P. indica* species. None of these species nor the European plantains are related to the plant that bears the plantain fruit/vegetable.

Cultivation
Plantains will grow in most soils and situations, but for the best leaves and seeds, give the European plantains moist soil in partial shade and the other psyllium species well-drained soil in sun. They will reach around 20–60cm (8–24in) in height and spread.

A History of Healing
Plantain leaves are the best first-aid remedy for a nettle sting (not dock – *Rumex* – as is sometimes thought, though that has some benefit), crushed and rubbed directly on the sting site. It is also traditionally used as a wound and bruise

healer, and is an ancient ingredient of poultices for drawing out stings, poison and abcesses, mentioned in the Anglo-Saxon herbal text *Lacnunga*. It also has anti-allergenic properties, and is a traditional hay-fever remedy. Astringent in nature, it was used for treating diarrhoea: Culpeper wrote that it 'prevails wonderfully against all torments or excoriations in the intestines or bowels'.

Psyllium seeds are high in fibre and gelatinous and are an effective aid to constipation. Surprisingly, they are also useful in cases of diarrhoea (several studies have proven this dual action), and are prescribed by herbalists for irritable bowel syndrome, ulcerative colitis and Crohn's disease. This general protective effect on the bowels is also thought to help the body rid itself of waste products and to alleviate haemorrhoids.

How to Use

Plantain leaves can be used fresh or dried in hot-water infusions as a digestive aid (add other herbs to improve the flavour). Combined with nettle and elderflower in a tisane, they can help relieve hay-fever symptoms. Use an infused oil for a balm for insect bites and nettle stings.

Soak psyllium seeds, available to buy from herbal suppliers, in water before taking with plenty of liquid.

PORTULACA OLERACEA

Purslane *Ma Chi Xian*

This fleshy-leaved annual retains the name given to it by Pliny the Elder, and has been used for centuries as food and medicine. A cultivated variety, *P. oleracea* subsp. *sativa*, is widely grown as a vegetable, especially in France, and is a principal ingredient of the Middle Easten salad fattoush.

Caution
Contraindicated as a remedy during pregnancy.

Cultivation
Purslane grows more or less all over the world. A half-hardy annual, it likes rich, moist but well-drained soil in full sun and will grow to around 30cm (12in) tall and 50cm (20in) wide. It is often found as a weed.

A History of Healing
Regarded as a global panacea in traditional Chinese medicine, purslane was first mentioned in a Chinese *Materia Medica* in 500 CE, and was used against fevers and toxins whether internal or as a result of stings or bites. The fleshy leaves are mucilaginous and soothing to the digestive system – they are given in TCM for gastrointestinal problems and appendicitis – as well as diuretic.

It is now known the plant contains relatively high levels of omega-3 fatty acids and is antibacterial.

Harvesting
Cut plants before flowering and use fresh or dry.

How to Use
Add fresh leaves to salads and other dishes.

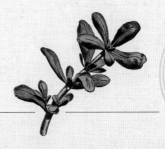

ORIGINS
Europe, Asia

PRIMULA VERIS

Cowslip *Paigle, fairy cups*

A tisty-tosty – a ball of threaded cowslip flower heads on a string – was part of an old country tradition of young people determining their true love or potential partner. The ball would be tossed between a group of girls or boys as they quickly spoke a list of possible candidates. The name spoken as the ball was dropped would be 'the one'.

Caution
Contraindicated during pregnancy and for people taking anticoagulant medication. Do not use if sensitive to aspirin.

Cultivation
Cowslips will naturalize in grass and woods. They prefer a drier soil in sun or partial shade. A hardy perennial, they will reach a height and spread of 15–20cm (6–8in).

A History of Healing
Cowslip tea and wine (a country drink widely made before habitat loss made cowslips rare in the wild) are both traditional drinks for calming the nerves and inducing sleep.

Parkinson recorded that country gentlewomen would also use the juice or flower water (it's not clear if it was infused or distilled) of cowslips 'to cleanse the skin from spots or discolourings therein, as also to take away the wrinckles thereof, and cause the skinne to become smooth and faire.' William Turner referred to this use as well but pointed out that it is entirely to 'make them fayre in the eyes of the worlde rather than in the eyes of God, whom they are not afryd to offend.'

Other old names for cowslip include herba paralysis and palsywort, and it was used from medieval times as an antispasmodic. This has led to interest in cowslips as having potential in the treatment of Parkinson's disease, epilepsy and asthma. The root is an expectorant, and has been used to slow the clotting of the blood, the aerial parts have a similar but weaker effect.

Foraging
Cowslips are extremely rare in the wild, and should not be picked. Cultivate plants in a garden to use instead, or buy the dried herb from herbal suppliers.

How to Use
A tea made from cowslip flowers can help induce a calm night's sleep and alleviate short-term restlessness; infused in honey or a syrup, they can have the same effect. Young leaves can be added to salads.

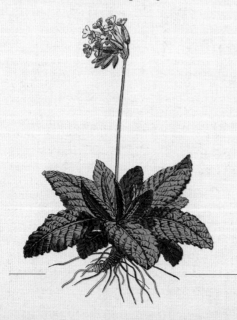

PRUNELLA VULGARIS

Selfheal *Heal-all, carpenter's herb, woundwort, Xia Cu Cao*

Although its common names allude to selfheal's properties as a wound healer, the name *Prunella* derives from the German *brunella*, from *bräune*, a quinsy or throat infection, which the plant also treats.

Cultivation
A creeping hardy perennial, growing to a maximum height of 50cm (20in), selfheal can be invasive in lawns but lovely in wildflower meadows. It prefers moist but well-drained soil in full sun or dappled shade.

A History of Healing
All the great herbals hold selfheal in high esteem as a wound herb. Gerard summarized it: 'There is not a better wounde herbe in the world', while Culpeper explained that, 'It is a special herb for inward and outward wounds,' and quoted a European proverb, 'That he needs neither physician nor surgeon that hath Self-heal and Sanicle [*Sanicula europaea*] to help himself.' It has

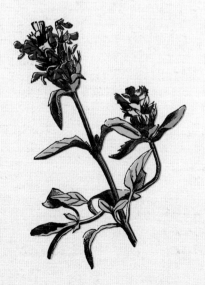

been proven to have antiviral properties, which would support Parkinson's claim that selfheal would not only help join together the lips of a green wound but also 'keepe the place from any further inconvenience'.

Modern herbalists value selfheal for its astringent and antioxidant properties, and find it beneficial in the case of sore throats as well as inflammatory bowel disease and internal bleeding. Elizabeth Blackwell recorded it as of use 'for all Inflammations and Ulcers in the Tongue, Jaws and Throat.' Traditional Chinese medicine uses the flowers (Xia Cu Cao) as a liver tonic and for complaints such as fevers, headaches, mumps and mastitis.

Harvesting
Cut long stems off the plants when in flower and hang to dry. Although selfheal can be easily foraged, a home-grown supply is a more reliable source.

How to Use
For minor cuts and grazes, the leaves of selfheal can be twisted and crushed before being applied directly to the (cleaned) site and secured with a plaster. Replace every eight hours or so. It can also be made into an infused oil and balm, especially for the treatment of haemorrhoids. A tea of the leaves or flowers may help heal inward wounds such as ulcers; added honey will help to soothe a sore throat.

PUERARIA MONTANA VAR. LOBATA (SYN. *P. LOBATA*, *P. THUNBERGIANA*)

Kudzu *Kudzu vine, Japanese arrowroot*

This deciduous vine is vigorous, hardy and will grow in most soils and situations, all of which made it an attractive plant to control soil erosion in 1930s America. However, it was soon realized that kudzu was a difficult-to-eradicate weed, growing up to 18m (59ft) in a single season.

Caution
Subject to legislation as an invasive species in some countries.

A History of Healing
The roots of the kudzu vine have been used since the 6th century BCE in traditional Chinese medicine as a remedy for muscle pain and stiffness, measles, headache, dizziness and diarrhoea. The flowers are used as a treatment for alcohol-related complaints, including hangovers. However, the root is thought to slow the liver's ability to process alcohol – modern research has shown the potential of kudzu in suppressing the appetite for alcohol.

Research has also shown that the roots contain isoflavones, oestrogenic compounds that may have potential in relieving menopausal symptoms, in particular associated memory loss.

How to Use
Kudzu can be used in cooking; the ground root is similar to arrowroot (see page 164).

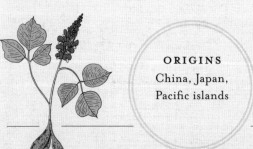

ORIGINS
China, Japan,
Pacific islands

REHMANNIA GLUTINOSA

Rehmannia *Di Huang, Chinese foxglove*

An important herb in traditional Chinese medicine, one of the 50 most used, rehmannia features in many herbal formulae.

Caution
Seek professional medical advice before using rehmannia during pregnancy. Contraindicated in the case of digestive problems.

Cultivation
A hardy perennial, rehmannia prefers full sun and will grow in a range of soil conditions, although damp situations may cause fungal rots. Rehmannia will grow up to 30cm (12in) in height and spread.

A History of Healing
Rehmannia is traditionally prepared in two different ways: fresh or dried roots (Sheng Di Huang) are used to treat hepatitis and protect the liver; its efficacy in this regard has been proven by clinical trials. Roots simmered in red wine (Shu Di Huang) are warming, a tonic to the kidneys, and used in cases of blood loss, such as heavy menstrual bleeding and childbirth.

How to Use
Dried whole or powdered root can be purchased from herbal suppliers, and decocted in red wine as a restorative drink for sufferers of anaemia and heavy periods.

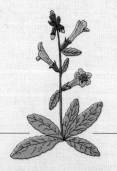

ORIGINS
North China

RHAMNUS

Cascara sagrada *European alder buckthorn*

Cascara sagrada (*R. purshiana*) is closely related to the European alder buckthorn (*R. frangula*, syn. *Frangula alnus*) and used in much the same way.

Caution
Berries are toxic. All parts are contraindicated during pregnancy and breastfeeding, and in cases of intestinal obstruction or excessive tension in the colon wall.

Cultivation
Well-drained soil in sun or partial shade will best suit cascara sagrada and alder buckthorn. They are hardy shrubs or small trees and can be grown as part of a mixed hedge.

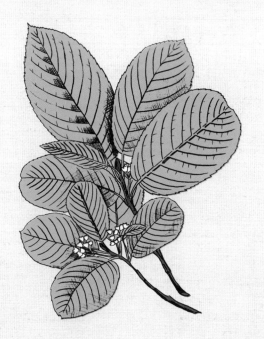

A History of Healing
The bark of all *Rhamnus* species contains compounds called anthraquinones, which have a laxative and purgative effect. Cascara sagrada was so popular a remedy in late 18th- and early 19th-century America that it was estimated around a hundred thousand trees were destroyed per year by indiscriminate bark stripping. It is most commonly taken as a decoction for chronic constipation, but also has benefits for other digestive and liver complaints, and is an overall digestive tonic. The bitter taste of the bark is also used, when applied externally, to deter nail biting.

Buckthorn (*R. cathartica*) has a more potent effect than either of the other species; it is mainly used today in veterinary medicine.

Harvesting
Harvested bark is left to dry for at least a year before using – fresh bark causes severe vomiting and griping.

How to Use
Cascara sagrada and buckthorn should only be taken after consulting a qualified herbalist and medical professional. Sea buckthorn (*Hippophae rhamnoides*) is not related to buckthorn and has nutritious edible berries.

RHEUM OFFICINALE

Chinese rhubarb *Da Huang*

Chinese rhubarb is the common name applied to both *R. officinale* and *R. palmatum*. They may be used interchangeably. Common rhubarb (*R. rhaponticum*) is not considered as medicinally beneficial.

Caution
Contraindicated during pregnancy, breastfeeding or menstruation, and in cases of intestinal obstruction, gout or kidney stones. Not suitable for children. The leaves are toxic.

Cultivation
Grow Chinese rhubarb in well-drained but moist and rich soil in full sun. It is a hardy perennial that can reach 2–3m (6½–10ft) tall and wide.

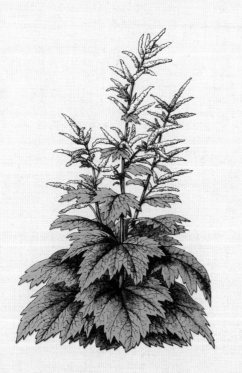

A History of Healing
Purgatives were an important part of the physician's or apothecary's toolkit, and so plants known to have strong laxative effects, like Chinese rhubarbs, were economically important, initially heavily traded between China and the West. Once European plant hunters managed to secure live plants, Chinese rhubarbs were extensively cultivated in physic gardens such as Chelsea and Edinburgh; historical maps of the latter show a large space dedicated to Chinese rhubarb.

The plant has been used as a remedy for constipation in traditional Chinese medicine for at least two thousand years, and is still used today in both herbal and conventional medicine for its laxative anthraquinone compounds. Conversely, smaller doses are astringent and can relieve diarrhoea by reducing intestinal irritation. Research shows antibacterial effects.

Harvesting
The rhizomes (roots) of six- to ten-year-old plants are dug up in autumn, after the leaves have begun to yellow, and dried before using.

How to Use
A small glass (around 100ml/½ cup) of a decoction of the dried root can be drunk in the evening to relieve occasional constipation.

ORIGINS
Arctic regions
of Europe,
North America
and Asia

RHODIOLA ROSEA

Roseroot *Rhodiola, golden root, Arctic root*

So-called because the roots of the plant are a pleasant shade of gold/pink, roseroot is an important adaptogen for subarctic countries such as Russia, Canada and Norway.

Caution
Can cause disturbed sleep and irritability; contraindicated for sufferers of manic and bipolar disorders.

Cultivation
Rhodiola is a fleshy perennial, fully hardy and growing to a mound of around 40cm (16in) tall and wide. It needs full sun and prefers well-drained soil.

A History of Healing
Rhodiola has traditionally been taken as an adaptogenic tonic to improve physical and mental endurance, helping users to better tolerate winter cold, high altitudes and to improve longevity and fertility. Small-scale trials have shown it to be effective in increasing the ability to resist mental and physical fatigue (the trial subjects were all doctors working night shifts) and also in treating mild depression, with fewer side-effects than conventional antidepressants. Russia made rhodiola an official medicine in 1969, to be used as an adaptogen and antidepressant.

Rhodiola works by supporting the health of neurotransmitters in the brain, preventing their decline under the influence of the stress hormone cortisol, and having a positive effect on the balance of hormones, promoting the 'happy hormones' serotonin and dopamine.

Harvesting
Rhodiola is cultivated on a small scale, but most herbal supplies are from wild plants, threatening the long-term survival of the species. Rhizomes (roots) are dried before use.

How to Use
Dried roots of home-grown plants can be prepared as a decoction or tincture and taken in small doses to support concentration and enhance physical endurance. Eat the leaves fresh in salads, although they are bitter, or preserve by fermenting into a sauerkraut-type pickle.

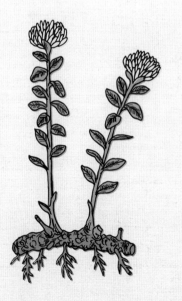

ROSA

Rose, apothecary's rose, dog rose and sweet briar

A plant that has more literary associations or a longer recorded history than the rose would be hard to find. It has sweetened the air around humankind for thousands of years, and is a symbol of loves both won and lost, bringing both joy and comfort. Unsurprisingly, the rose also has a long association with herbal remedies, used both for its petals and hips. The young leaves are astringent and can be taken as an infusion, but they are not much used today.

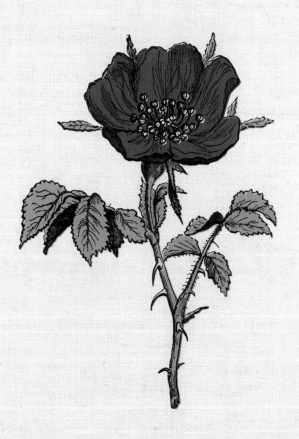

Caution
Rosehips contain minute, highly irritant hairs that should not be ingested, so be sure to process the hips correctly when making jellies, ketchup or syrup.

'A Rose by Any Other Name'
In theory, any rose can be used for its petals or hips, provided they have not been sprayed with chemical fertilizers or pesticides, but some species are better than others. In general, more ancient species will be closest to those used by herbalists in the past, and the petals more delicate than those of the modern hybrids. For petals, choose the most fragrant species and cultivars, notably the damask roses *R.* × *damascena* and *R. gallica*, which is most commonly found in cultivation as *R. gallica* var. *officinalis* (the apothecary's rose), or *R.* 'Kazanlik', the variety most used for producing rose-water in Bulgaria. For a year-round supply of petals, try growing *R.* × *odorata* 'Bengal Crimson' in a sheltered position – at the Chelsea Physic Garden, a specimen of this rose is in flower every day, except following a severe pruning to keep its vigorous growth in check.

Hips can be gathered from cultivated or wild roses. Hedgerow roses are likely to be the dog rose (*R. canina*) or sweet briar (*R. rubiginosa*). *Rosa rugosa* hips are large and fleshy, and the petals well fragranced too, but it is subject to legal restrictions as an invasive plant.

Cultivation

Roses, in general, prefer rich, moist but well-drained soil in sun. Prune according to guidance for each species, removing dead and diseased wood, and clearing away any fallen leaves infected with blackspot. Hedgerow roses such as the dog rose will scramble up to 3m (10ft) high and wide, *R. damascena* can get to 2m (6½ft), and *R. gallica* around 1m (3ft) in height and spread.

A History of Healing

The Ancient Romans were inordinately fond of roses, scattering the petals around their homes and streets. The Emperor Nero lavished roses on his festivities, even ordering fountains to run with rose-water. To fragrance houses (and disguise odours), roses continued to be popular from the Elizabethan era onwards, either as a strewing herb or mixed into a potpourri.

Rose-water and oil, first distilled around 1000 CE by Avicenna, an Arab physician, was used as a personal perfume, and it was said to be the favourite of Henry VIII. Cold cream, the moisturizing lotion that graced many a dressing table of old, was originally known as 'ointment of roses' because it is prepared using rose oil and rose-water. Rose continues to be used in perfumes and cosmetics today, though it is often now synthetic or extracted from pelargonium species (see page 181) because pure rose oil is extremely expensive. Known as otto, or attar,

ROSEHIP SYRUP

Whizz 100g (1¼ cups) of clean, de-stalked rosehips in a food processor or chop them very finely. Bring 160ml (⅔ cup) of water to the boil in a small, lidded saucepan, then add the hips. Bring back to the boil then remove from the heat and leave to stand for 20 minutes. Strain through a jelly bag or muslin-lined sieve (do not squeeze or press the pulp, just leave it until it stops dripping) and set aside the juice. Return the pulp to the pan with 120ml (½ cup) water and bring to the boil. Remove from the heat and leave to stand for another 20 minutes, rinsing clean the bag/muslin in the meantime. Strain again, as above, and discard the pulp. Combine the two sets of juice with 60g (⅓ cup) of sugar (any type) in a clean saucepan, stirring to dissolve. Bring to the boil and continue boiling for 4 minutes then pour into small warm, sterilized bottles. Keeps up to one year unopened; once open, store in the fridge and use within two weeks. Shake the bottle before using.

of roses, rose oil is said to lift the spirits and be mildly sedative when used in aromatherapy.

Rose petals are edible, and were used in food from Roman to medieval times; until the arrival of vanilla in Europe as the universal flavouring and sweetener, it was rose-water that gave a fragrance to cakes and other foods.

Roses were also widely esteemed in medieval medicine as a remedy for depression, and have historically also been used to treat sore throats and mild digestive complaints. Rose petals are said to have a balancing effect on the hormones, and can help to lift and calm the mood in the case of premenstrual and menopausal irritation. To soothe a headache, a rose cold compress was traditionally used. Mrs Grieve wrote in her herbal that, 'Rose Vinegar, a specific on the Continent for headache caused by hot sun, is prepared by steeping dried rose petals in best distilled vinegar, which should not be boiled. Cloths or linen rags are soaked in the liquid and applied to the head.'

Rosehips have a tannin content that makes them effective against diarrhoea, as recorded by Culpeper: 'The fruits of the wild briar, which are called Hips, being thoroughly ripe, and made into a conserve with sugar, beside the pleasantness of the taste, doth gently bind the belly.' During the Second World War, when naval blockades prevented the import of citrus fruit, a botanist at Kew Gardens determined that the dog rose had the highest vitamin C content, and a large foraging endeavour was initiated. Thousands of tons of hips were gathered and processed into syrup to give to children, a practice that continued every winter into the 1960s.

Modern research shows that vitamin C is needed by the body in the production of collagen, which is not just a wrinkle-plumper but also an essential component of tendons and ligaments, so rosehips could have some application in cases of muscle pain and rheumatism.

ROSES ARE RED…

There are many legends surrounding the origins of the red rose, the universal flower of love and passion. They include a white rose that blushed on receiving a kiss from Eve; that it was stained red with Venus's blood as she searched for her lover Adonis; or that it was stained with red wine spilt from Cupid's cup.

Dog roses are said to get their name both from their use to cure the bite of a wild dog, and from a corruption of dag, from 'dagger', referring to the thorns.

A rose suspended over the dining table signifies that the evening's conversation should be kept in confidence – plaster ceiling ornaments are called a rose to this day.

Harvesting and Foraging
Pick rose petals when they are young and fragrant, to use fresh or to dry – avoid any that might have been sprayed by chemical fertilizers or pesticides. Rosehips appear in late summer to autumn but wait to pick them until after the first frost, when they will be softer.

How to Use

Infuse rose petals in hot water for an uplifting, fragrant tisane (or mix with other herbs to add flavour). They can also be infused in honey, or made into rose petal jam. Infused in vinegar they can be used as a hair rinse or cold compress for headaches; infused in oil, they make a relaxing massage oil. Sprinkle dried and ground petals over food, mix with other spices for a fragrant rub for meat and vegetables, or with honey to soothe a sore throat.

Rose-water is made by distilling the petals and is best left to professionals. Most commercial rose-water is a by-product of the rose oil industry, though a Welsh rose-water producer makes rose-water from the first distillation of the petals, which gives it a high oil content as well. Rose-water can be used for cooking and cocktails, as a facial toner, or to mist onto the body, to refresh and calm. Attar of roses can be diluted in a carrier oil for massage.

Rosehips can be made into syrup (see page 197), for taking by the teaspoonful or diluted in hot water, added to hedgerow jellies and ketchups, such as those with hawthorn berries (see page 114) and elderberries (see page 210), or dried and powdered. If using hips in syrups or preserves, catch the irritant hairs by straining them through a fine muslin or jelly bag.

To make rosehip powder, halve and scoop out the seeds from the hips and then dry the flesh. Once dried, whizz to a powder in a food processor or spice grinder. Sprinkle the powder over porridge, cereals, puddings and savoury dishes.

MRS GRIEVE'S ROSE PETAL SANDWICHES

'Put a layer of Red Rose-petals in the bottom of a jar or covered dish, put in 4oz. [115g] of fresh butter. Cover with a thick layer of rose-petals. Cover closely and leave in a cool place overnight. The more fragrant the roses, the finer the flavour imparted. Cut bread in thin strips or circles, spread each with the perfumed butter and place several petals from fresh Red Roses between the slices, allowing edges to show. Violets or Clover blossoms may be used in place of Roses'.

RUBUS

Raspberry and blackberry

Raspberries (*Rubus idaeus*) and blackberries (*R. fruticosus*) are both delicious and nutritious fruits that can be added to the diet, but the leaves have a history of herbal use as well.

Caution
Do not take raspberry leaf tea during pregnancy, except for the last few weeks. Blackberries are subject to control as an invasive plant in some countries.

Cultivation
Both species will need supporting stakes and tying into wires as the canes are long and floppy. They prefer rich soil and full sun. Remove old stems after fruiting.

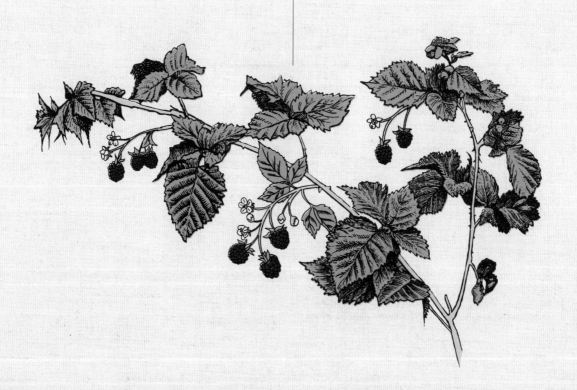

A History of Healing

Most mothers will be aware of raspberry leaf tea as a gentle herbal remedy traditionally used in the last few weeks of pregnancy in the belief it will ease childbirth. Research is still ongoing into the exact effects raspberry extracts have on the womb and menstrual symptoms, but it is thought that they help to tone the muscles of the uterus so that contractions will be more effective.

Dioscorides recommended blackberries as a sore throat remedy, and both raspberry and blackberry leaves are still used today as an astringent gargle or mouthwash. Superstition attributes blackberry plants with magical properties when they arch and root at both ends – it is said that children with hernias who ran beneath would be cured.

The fruit of both species are antioxidant and vitamin-rich.

Harvesting

Wild raspberries are preferred for therapeutic use, but home-grown plants can also be used. Pick the leaves as required to use fresh, and/or dry or freeze them. Fruits can be picked when ripe. It is said that blackberries picked after Michaelmas (29 September) will bring bad luck, because the Devil has spat on them – and it is certainly true that the first frosts around this time will cause the fruits to rot.

How to Use

Infuse the leaves of blackberry plants to use as a gargle or mouthwash for ulcers or sore throats. Raspberry leaves infused in hot water can be drunk to help childbirth but only in the last few weeks of pregnancy and during labour.

ORIGINS
Northern
temperate and
Arctic regions

RUMEX ACETOSA

Sorrel *Common sorrel, garden sorrel, sour grabs, cuckoo-sorrow*

The *Rumex* genus includes docks and sorrels. Some wild species, such as sheep's sorrel (*R. acetosella*), are favoured by foragers for their tangy leaves; other sorrels can be cultivated as lemon-flavoured salad herbs, especially the attractive red-veined variety *R. sanguineus* var. *sanguineus*.

Cultivation
Sorrel prefers moist soil in sun or partial shade. A hardy perennial, it will reach around 40cm (16in) in height and spread. Divide and replant older plants that run to seed too quickly to refresh them.

A History of Healing
Parkinson wrote of sorrel's cooling and drying qualities for 'any inflammation and heate of bloud…and to refresh the overspent spirits'. The roots and seeds were prepared as decoctions, and the leaves made into a juice,

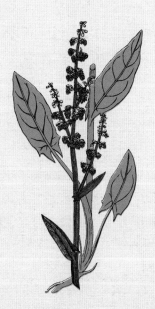

often used for ulcers and sores on the skin. The leaves are rich in vitamins A and C, and were widely used as a cure for scurvy. They are also slightly bitter, so have a mild stimulating effect on the digestion.

Sheep's sorrel is an ingredient of the Native American anticancer remedy essiac, which also includes burdock (see page 86) and slippery elm (see page 234). The remedy was observed by a Canadian nurse in the early 20th century and she developed a proprietary formula, still available today as a powder and tea. Although anecdotal evidence is positive, no well-designed clinical trials have yet proven that it has any positive anticancer effects, and it may produce unpleasant side-effects.

Harvesting
Pick the fresh leaves as needed throughout the year. Pick the flowers then cut off the flowering stalk to prevent it seeding all over the garden and to encourage fresh leaves.

How to Use
Add the fresh leaves (and flowers) to salads. The leaves can also be used to make a green sauce for fish, and substituted in part for other herbs in home-made pesto. Finely chopped with wild garlic, chives, parsley or other herbs, they make a delicious garnish for pasta and risotto dishes.

ORIGINS
Europe, North
Africa, North
Turkey,
the Azores

RUSCUS ACULEATUS

Butcher's broom *Knee holly*

Butcher's broom was indeed used as a brush to sweep the floor of butchers' shops until the 20th century. Its other common name refers to the fact that it is a low-growing, prickly evergreen shrub, although it has no actual botanical relationship with holly (*Ilex*). It is a curious-looking plant: what looks like the leaves are actually part of the branches, and the flowers and berries are borne in the centre of these.

Caution
Contraindicated if suffering from high blood pressure/hypertension.

Cultivation
Butcher's broom is an evergreen shrub growing to around 1m (3ft) in height and spread. It is fully hardy and prefers well-drained soil in sun or shade.

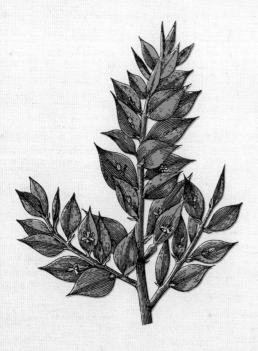

A History of Healing
Butcher's broom was mentioned as a remedy for kidney stones, as it promoted the flow of urine, and also as a stimulant to menstruation. The plant is now known to contain saponins, which have a similar effect to that of diosgenin from wild yam (see page 123), causing the contraction of the veins (and arteries, to a lesser extent). This contributes to their use as a traditional remedy for haemorrhoids and varicose veins, taken both internally and applied externally.

Culpeper had this helpful advice on preparing the roots: 'The more of the root you boil, the stronger will the decoction be; it works no ill-effects, yet I hope you have wit enough to give the strongest decoction to the strongest bodies.'

Harvesting
Both the roots and the shoots can be used. Cut and eat the youngest shoots like asparagus, in spring; cut the branches in late spring. Lift the roots in autumn and dry before use.

How to Use
Prepare the dried roots as a decoction to drink or spray directly onto the legs when suffering from varicose veins. Infuse fresh or dried branches and use in the same way. Taken internally, the infusion can be mildly laxative.

SALIX ALBA

Willow *White willow*

There are many willow species, many of them beautiful ornamental trees, but the white willow and goat willow (*Salix caprea*) are considered the most useful therapeutically. All over their native habitat, willows have a herbal tradition of being used for pain relief and, although it is meadowsweet with its old botanical name of *Spiraea*, that gives its name to aspirin, 'salicylic acid' derives from the genus name *Salix*. A wand made of willow was said to help a Druid or witch deter evil, while white willow today is used to make cricket bats.

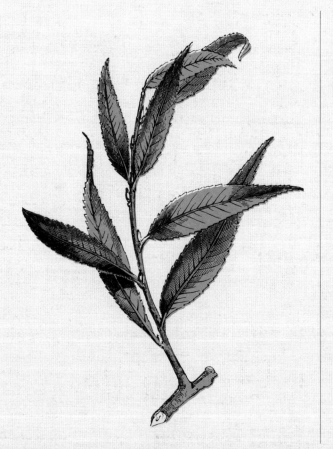

Caution
Contraindicated for people allergic or sensitive to aspirin (salicylates) and during pregnancy and breastfeeding. Not suitable for children.

Cultivation
Willows are often seen growing along riverbanks – they prefer moist (wet, even) soil in full sun. They will grow to large trees, 25m (82ft) tall, but can be pollarded. Willows are deciduous and fully hardy.

A History of Healing
Over 2,500 years ago, the Ancient Greek physician Hippocrates recommended willow as a remedy to relieve pain and fever, and it was recorded as being used as an antirheumatic on Sumerian clay tablets 3,500 years before that. Although Culpeper made no mention of any pain-relieving qualities, he did recommend a decoction of the 'leaves or bark in wine' as a hair rinse against dandruff. The leaves boiled in wine could also, according to Culpeper, stay 'the heat of lust in man or woman' – extinguishing

it permanently 'if it be long used'. In North America the native willow, *S. nigra*, is used for the same anaphrodisiac purpose. Willow extracts are also used in cosmetic products.

In 1838, two years after the compound was first isolated from meadowsweet (see page 132), salicylic acid was isolated from salicin, a compound found in willow bark. However, the first clinical trials proving willow bark's ability to reduce pain and fever were actually conducted in 1763 by the Reverend Edward Stone in Oxfordshire. Inspired by the Doctrine of Signatures (see page 19), he noted that the willow tree often grew in swampy ground associated with fever and malaria. He tested willow bark on patients with fever to great effect, and reported his findings to the Royal Society. As salicylic acid does not thin the blood or cause digestive side-effects as aspirin can, it is the subject of much current scientific interest. Tests so far have proven it is anti-inflammatory, giving it potential in treating joint pain. Herbalists often combine willow bark with St John's wort (see page 146) and cramp bark (see page 243) in a decoction for aching muscles. Willow's potential in reducing fever – and the associated sweating – also means it has applications for menopausal hot flushes and night sweats.

Harvesting
Pick the leaves through the spring and summer to use fresh or dried. Collect the bark in the summer – cut young branches and strip off the bark to use fresh or dried.

How to Use
Use a decoction or tincture of the bark for general pain and fever relief, and also to help alleviate pain from joints and arthritis. The bark can also be infused in oil to massage into the affected joints externally.

ORIGINS
Mediterranean,
North Africa

SALVIA OFFICINALIS

Sage *Garden sage*

Although the medieval adage, 'Why should a man die when he has sage in his garden?' is something of an overstatement of its medicinal properties, it does remind us to look to the garden – rather than the pharmacy – when in need of a tonic or remedy for a minor ill. Varieties of common sage, such as purple sage 'Purpurascens' and 'Kew Gold', a yellow-leaved dwarf form, can be used interchangeably with the species. Sage flowers are rich in nectar, so they are an excellent plant for attracting and helping bees.

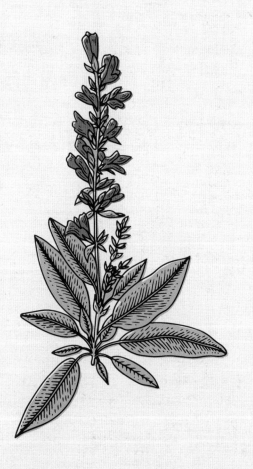

Caution
Eat only as a culinary herb (that is, do not use any preparations or sage remedies) during pregnancy and while breastfeeding, and in cases of epilepsy. Toxic if taken in excess or over a prolonged period.

Cultivation
Sage forms an evergreen bush around 60–75cm (2–2½ft) high and 1m (3ft) wide. Cut back regularly to keep it from becoming straggly, and replace with a new plant every four to six years. It prefers full sun and a well-drained soil, and is hardy unless the winter is particularly wet.

A History of Healing

Sage has distinct and proven antibacterial, antiseptic and anti-inflammatory properties, and has long been associated with treating sore throats, mouth ulcers and infected gums. Culpeper wrote that, 'The juice of Sage taken in warm water, helps a hoarseness and a cough.' The fresh leaves were also used to rub the teeth and gums before the advent of toothbrushes. It is also stimulating to the digestion as a bitter herb, helping to relieve wind and bloating.

Traditionally viewed as a drying herb, sage has been used to decrease the milk of breastfeeding mothers during the weaning process and also to reduce night sweats, especially of the menopause. Modern studies have investigated this latter application with some trials reporting positive results.

The phrases 'sage advice' and 'old sage' refer to this herb, which was renowned for its benefits to the brain and memory. Gerard wrote that sage was 'singularly good for the head and brain and quickeneth the nerves and memory.' Several modern studies have shown that sage can improve both learning and memory – with distinct possibilities for it as a remedy for Alzheimer's disease – possibly due to compounds present in the plant that protect the breakdown of neurotransmitters in the brain.

Clary sage (*S. sclarea*), also known as clear eye, has a long history as a remedy for eye problems, but it is most commonly used by herbalists today for its oestrogenic activity. It is a tonic herb during menopause and premenstrual tension, as well as being generally beneficial to the digestion; Elizabeth Blackwell wrote that, 'Infused in wine it comforts a cold Windy stomach.'

Harvesting

Pick fresh leaves as required. Cut branches in mid-summer, to dry.

How to Use

Drink a tisane of sage for a sore throat, as a memory aid and digestive tonic, and to relieve night sweats – it is an acquired taste, so combine with other herbs, if preferred – or gargle with it (see page 55).

Combine sage with other herbs to make a herb butter (finely chop the herbs, mash into the butter and reshape into a log), to use in sandwiches or other dishes. Parkinson wrote that, 'The use of Sage in the Moneth of May, with butter, Parsley and some salt, is very frequent in our Country to continue good health to the body.'

Dried leaves combined with dried wormwood leaves (see page 88) and put into fabric sachets make an effective moth repellent when placed in drawers and wardrobes. Chia seeds, from *S. hispanica*, a related species native to Mexico and northern South America, are eaten for their high fibre content and essential fatty acids. They can be sprinkled over sweet and savoury foods, or soaked and cooked to make a porridge or dessert. Soaked seeds diluted with lemon juice, sugar and water form a refreshing drink (also known as chia).

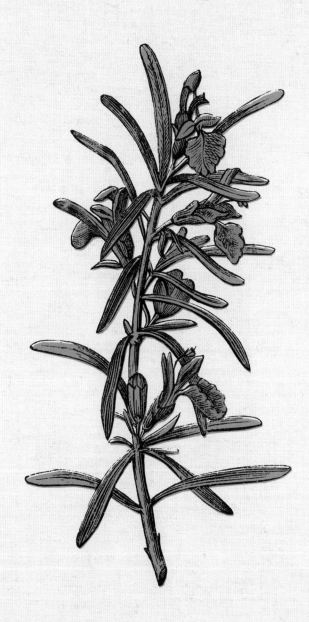

ORIGINS
Mediterranean

SALVIA ROSMARINUS (SYN. ROSMARINUS OFFICINALIS)

Rosemary

Rosemary is said to stimulate the memory and is traditionally used as a plant to symbolize remembrance of lost loved ones. Ophelia refers to this among other flower meanings when mourning her father in Shakespeare's *Hamlet*:
'There's rosemary, that's for remembrance; pray,
love, remember: and there's pansies, that's for thoughts'

Cultivation
Rosemary prefers well-drained soil and full sun, growing up to 1m (3ft) tall and wide in these conditions. It is evergreen, and hardy unless waterlogged in winter wet.

A History of Healing
In Ancient Greece it was the custom to smell a sprig of rosemary before undertaking an exam – a custom that continues to this day in Greece, although the herb is more often burned in the home, a practice that Elizabeth Blackwell considered 'good to Sweeten the Air'. Modern research has proven that smelling the essential oil can indeed enhance the brain's activity and improve the memory.

Rosemary is considered a general warming, tonic herb for longevity, low mood and nervous tension. It is thought stimulating to the circulation especially, encouraging blood flow to the brain and relieving headaches. Culpeper wrote that a decoction either drunk or bathed onto the head would relieve 'all other cold diseases of the head and brain, as the giddiness or swimmings therein, drowsiness or dullness of the mind and senses'. Blackwell reported that rosemary was 'accounted good for affections of the Head & Nerves. It strengthens ye Sight and Memory.'

The stimulating effects of rosemary are also traditionally used externally both to relieve muscle aches and also as a hair and scalp tonic, to help stimulate hair growth and reduce the flakiness of the scalp. It can also brighten the complexion when included in facial creams.

Harvesting
Cut fresh sprigs as needed; cut whole branches to dry in mid-spring and/or mid-summer.

How to Use
A hot-water infusion makes a refreshing drink that can uplift the mood and strengthen the mind and body, or simply rub a sprig between the fingers when in the garden, or cut some to have at your desk. Use the rosemary hair tonic (see page 64).

SAMBUCUS NIGRA

Elder *Elderflower, elderberry, pipe tree*

Steeped in folklore and superstition, elder trees grow in most urban
scrubland and parks as well as rural hedgerows. As such, it is usually possible
to find good trees from which to forage, but for a guaranteed supply of fresh
flowers and berries, you could grow your own.

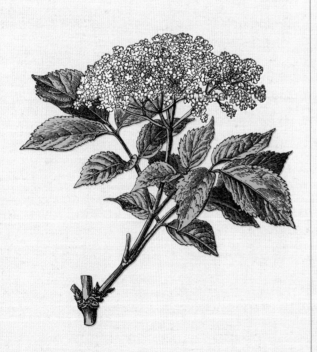

Cultivation
Elder grows best in rich soil in full sun or partial
shade. It can reach up to 10m (33ft) tall and 6m
(20ft) wide; pruning can keep it to size but do
not prune too hard, as it flowers on older wood.

A History of Healing
The flowers are a traditional remedy for
fevers, inducing sweating. The flowers are also
helpful in protecting against the symptoms of
hay fever, traditionally combined with yarrow
and peppermint in infusions for that purpose
and taken for a month before hay-fever season
starts. In her herbal Mrs Grieve reported that
the flowers were sometimes preserved in salt –
pickled – as well as dried.

Elderberries are rich in flavonoids,
antioxidants and vitamins A and C, and have
been used down the ages as a preventative tonic
against the winter onslaught of cold viruses.
Research has now shown that, as well as their
nutritional benefit, they may also help by
preventing viruses from attaching to the cells of
the nose and throat, enabling the body to expel
or digest them without getting infected.

Historically, elder leaves and bark were
also used by physicians – the bark for purging,

and the leaves infused in oils and balms for external bruising and chilblains – but they are less popular now, not least because the purging effect is so violent. The leaves are thought to deter insects, and an 18th-century gardening remedy made an infusion of the leaves to spray over kitchen garden crops. Jelly ears, a fungus that is prone to grow upon the bark of elder trees, is eaten in China and reputed to cure inflammations of the throat.

ANCIENT ELDER

The elder tree is known as the people's medicine chest, a herb with the potential to heal most minor complaints, and as such many superstitions have arisen around it. Many Scandinavian traditions attribute it with magical properties: it is said that the Mother Elder (Hylde-Moer) will curse any wood taken from her trees without permission; were a cradle to be made from elder wood, she would follow the family and pull at the baby's legs until it was removed. Gypsy tradition is never to burn elder wood – either from fear of the old folklore or because it was also reputed to be the wood of Christ's cross. An early medieval rhyme, using a contemporary common name for elder, the bour tree, runs:

'Bour tree, bour tree, crooked rong
Never straight and never strong
Ever bush and never tree
Since our lord was nailed on thee'

Demonstrating how the oldest superstitions easily get twisted and corrupted down the ages, elder was, conversely, also used to ward off evil. In William Coles' 1656 *Art of Simpling,* he wrote that, 'in order to prevent witches from entering their houses, the common people used to gather *Elder leaves* on the last day of April and affix them to their doors and windows.' Wands made from elder wood are held to be particularly powerful, a superstition repeated in the Harry Potter series of books, and a bewitched person should be given a bough of elder to break the spell.

More prosaically, the spongy middle of the elder stem can be easily removed, and it was used to make musical pipes in ancient civilizations, and pop-guns for country boys in Culpeper's time.

The name elder derives from the Anglo-Saxon *aeld*, which means to blow up fire – presumably the hollow stems were blown through to kindle the flames from a safe distance.

Foraging and Harvesting

Look for the frothy white flowers of elder in late spring, and return for the berries in early to mid-autumn. Leave some flowers on the bush or there won't be any berries; birds also love the berries, so while you need to harvest them before they disappear, leave some for the wildlife. Elderflowers are best harvested when around a third of the buds on the spray are still closed and the whole head is creamy white with no hint of browning petals. Elderberries are ready when they turn from green to a deep purple – take care, as the juice will stain. Both flowers and berries can be dried, and the berries can also be frozen to use later. Berries must be cooked or dried before eating to remove toxins that can cause vomiting. Ask permission of and/ or apologize to the Hylde-Moer (also known as Lady Ellhorn) at your discretion!

How to Use

The flowers can be preserved in a cordial (see page 133), which is then drunk diluted with hot or cold water, or dried flowers can be infused in hot water, both of which make a refreshing drink that will help to reduce fevers and provide some protection against cold and flu viruses and hay fever. Infusions of the flowers can induce perspiration, so drink with plenty of fluids. Berries can be cooked fresh, preserved in a syrup (see below) or vinegar, or frozen to cook at a later date – try a handful in an apple crumble. Either way, they will provide a boost to the immune system to protect against or to speed recovery from colds and flu.

ELDERBERRY SYRUP

Have this neat by the spoonful or dilute into hot water for a delicious winter drink. It can also be stirred into cocktails and home-made lemonade.

2kg (4½lb) elderberry sprays, washed

1 unwaxed orange, zest only

2 cinnamon sticks

1 tbsp cloves

5cm (2in) piece fresh ginger (alternatively, add other spices such as 1 tbsp cardamom pods or 4 star anise – experiment to find your favourite combination)

unrefined granulated or caster sugar

lemon juice

Separate the berries from the stalks using the tines of a fork and put into a saucepan. Add water to cover, then stir in the orange zest, spices and ginger. Bring to the boil and simmer, covered, until the berries are soft (around 30 minutes). Remove the pan from the heat and use a potato masher to squash the juice from the berries before straining through a jelly bag or muslin-lined sieve into a measuring jug. Squeeze out as much juice as possible from the skins, then discard the pulp. For every 500ml (2 cups) of juice, add 450g (2¼ cups) sugar and the juice of one lemon, mixing them into the juice in a large pan. (For extra spice, fish out the spices from the initial mix and add them back into the juice pan.) Bring to the boil, stirring to dissolve the sugar, then simmer for 10–15 minutes to thicken it. Strain, if necessary, and pour into warm, sterilized bottles; seal and label. Will keep for a year unopened; once opened, store in the refrigerator.

ORIGINS
Southern Europe,
North Africa

SATUREJA

Summer savory and winter savory

Summer savory (*Satureja hortensis*) and its winter cousin *S. montana* are both used as culinary herbs, with a distinct peppery note. The winter form is more bitter than the summer.

Cultivation
Well-drained or even dry soil in full sun will suit the savories best. They will grow to 20–30cm (8–12in) high and wide. Summer savory is an annual, winter savory a hardy perennial.

A History of Healing
Galen and Dioscorides considered winter savory to have heating and drying properties, and it was used against diarrhoea. Centuries later it was taken by European colonists to North America

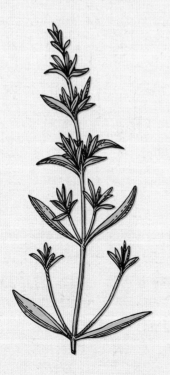

for that very purpose. Culpeper recommended everyone to 'keep it dry by you all the year, if you love yourself and your ease.'

Both the savory species are stimulating to the digestion, carminative and useful in the case of bronchial infections (similar in effect to thyme, see page 227). It is now known that this is due to the presence of the essential oil thymol in the leaves, which is antibacterial. Their carminative activity makes them ideal to use in bean dishes, and they are popular herbs in Italy for that purpose. Summer savory is a traditional flavouring for sausages in Germany.

Tips for Growing
To crop fresh summer savory in winter, sow seeds in early autumn and grow in a greenhouse or cold frame, or pull up the whole plant in summer to dry (this should be done as it flowers, so denies the wildlife a feast). Cut back winter savory in spring to encourage new bushy growth.

How to Use
Infuse the fresh leaves in hot water for a digestive tonic and healing tea for colds and flu. Summer savory leaves are now considered therapeutically weaker than winter savory, though Culpeper believed the opposite.

ORIGINS
Northeast China,
Japan

SCHISANDRA CHINENSIS

Schisandra *Magnolia vine, Wu Wei Zi*

The 'five-flavoured herb' was first brought to Western botanical and physic gardens in the 1850s, but was mentioned in Chinese medical texts almost two thousand years earlier. The 'five flavours' refer to the sweet peel and sour pulp of the fruit, and the bitter, salty and acrid flavours of the seeds thought to correspond to the five principal elemental energies of traditional Chinese medicine.

Caution
Seek professional medical advice before using schisandra if you are taking other medication, as it could negatively interact with them. Excessive doses can cause heartburn.

Cultivation
This hardy deciduous climber needs rich, moist but well-drained soil and will grow in sun or partial shade, reaching up to 8m (26ft) tall. To have fruits, it will be necessary to grow both a male and a female plant.

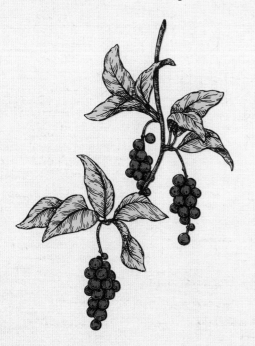

A History of Healing
Schisandra is a tonic herb, strengthening and toning the major organs, and considered an adaptogen that is good for gently increasing energy levels and stamina, and improving concentration. In Russia it has been used to treat mental health disorders as the berries are thought to be mildly antidepressant, also helping in cases of disturbed sleep. Schisandra is known to contain various compounds that protect the liver and help treat liver conditions such as hepatitis. However, its most widely used attribute in China is as a sexual tonic and it is thought to improve sexual desire and stamina.

Harvesting
Pick the berries after the first frosts. They are traditionally dried in the sun before using, but drying indoors will suffice.

How to Use
Prepare dried berries as a decoction, which can be taken as a general adaptogenic tonic and to improve the sex drive, or in the short term to relieve a cough.

SCROPHULARIA NODOSA

Common figwort *Knotted figwort*

This plant is known as *herbe du siège* in France, a name that dates back to the 1627–8 siege by Cardinal Richelieu's troops of La Rochelle during the English-supported Huguenot uprising in early 17th-century France. Starving, the besieged were reduced to eating the tuberous roots of figwort to survive.

Caution
Contraindicated in cases of heart conditions.

Cultivation
Figwort prefers moist or even wet soil in sun or partial shade. It is a hardy perennial and will grow to around 40cm (16in) in height and spread.

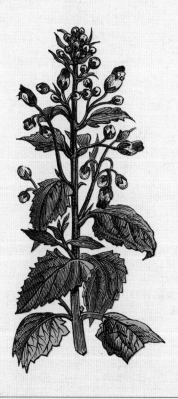

A History of Healing
'A better remedy there cannot be for the king's evil,' wrote Culpeper. The king's evil is an old name for scrofula, the condition in which the lymph nodes of the neck form hard, bulging lumps after being infected with tuberculosis. It is thought that the Doctrine of Signatures (see page 19) therefore pointed in the direction of figwort as a cure, though whether it is because the flowers resemble the throat or the roots resemble the lumpy glands is not clear. As well as scrofula, figwort was used in treating all manner of tumours and swellings: as Culpeper put it, 'any other knobs, kernel, bunches, or wens growing in the flesh wheresoever; and for the haemorrhoids'. It was taken both internally and applied externally as a poultice. It is now known that the leaves contain wound-healing compounds. Herbalists also recommend it as an internal cleansing herb and a poultice for chronic skin diseases.

Harvesting
Pick the leaves fresh and/or cut the whole plant when it is flowering and dry it.

How to Use
Infuse fresh or dried aerial parts in hot water for a cleansing drink – the leaves have an unpleasant aroma, so combine it with more palatable herbs, if desired.

ORIGINS
China, Japan,
Mongolia
(*S. baicalensis*);
North America
(*S. lateriflora*)

SCUTELLARIA

Skullcap *Baical skullcap, helmet flower, Huang Quin* (S. baicalensis); *Virginian skullcap, mad dog* (S. lateriflora)

The use of *Scutellaria baicalensis* (baical skullcap) in traditional Chinese medicine dates back to at least the 2nd century CE. Its North American native counterpart, *S. lateriflora*, also has a long tradition of use, though for quite different complaints. *Scutellaria altissima* is sometimes sold as Virginian skullcap, too, but this is a larger and more floriferous species, so check the identification before using.

Caution
Excessive doses of *S. lateriflora* can cause serious side-effects to the nervous system – take only under professional supervision and never during pregnancy.

Cultivation
Baical skullcap needs a well-drained to dry soil and will reach 40cm (16in) tall and 30cm (12in) wide, while Virginian skullcap prefers damp soils and will grow to a height of around 60cm (2ft) with a spread of around 40cm (16in). Both are hardy perennials and will grow in sun or partial shade.

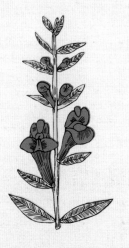

A History of Healing
In TCM, baical skullcap roots are considered a cold herb, and are used to treat hot conditions such as dysentery, urinary infections and fevers. It is known to have anti-inflammatory, antioxidant and anti-allergenic effects, mostly due to a high percentage of flavonoids in the roots. Clinical studies have shown encouraging results in treating obesity and some cancers.

A 19th-century treatment for rabies, Virginian skullcap was used by the indigenous population for menstrual problems. Mrs Grieve wrote in *A Modern Herbal* that 'many cases of hydrophobia have been cured by this remedy alone'. It was also used to alleviate stress and nervous conditions, though excessive use can cause giddiness, seizures or stupor.

Harvesting
Lift the roots of three- to four-year-old plants of baical skullcap in spring or autumn to use fresh or dried. The leaves of Virginian skullcap can be picked to use fresh or dried.

How to Use
Virginian skullcap can be taken in moderation as a nerve tonic and for the short-term relief of stress, but consult a herbalist first. Baical skullcap can be decocted for a remedy for chesty coughs and fever, or made into a tincture for hay-fever relief.

SERENOA REPENS
(SYN. S. SERRULATA, SABAL SERRULATA)

Saw palmetto

A wild plant found in sand dunes from South Carolina to Texas, saw palmetto is currently being researched for its potential in treating enlarged prostate glands.

Caution
Contraindicated during pregnancy and breastfeeding. Do not take if also taking hormonal drugs or in cases of hormone-dependent cancers.

Cultivation
Saw palmetto is an evergreen, shrubby palm tree growing to 2–4m (6½–13ft) in height. It spreads indefinitely through creeping, suckering rhizomes. It prefers damp or wet soil in sun or dappled shade and needs a minimum temperature of 7°C (45°F).

A History of Healing
The nutty vanilla-flavoured fruits of the saw palmetto were an important foodstuff for the indigenous tribespeople of Florida, the native habitat of the herb. Those who ate them noticed they had a sedative effect and caused a general improvement in physical condition, which was remarked upon in their animals as well. When the European colonists noticed this, they too began to eat the berries. They are taken as a strengthening tonic to this day, although the berries are now used primarily for their diuretic effect, general healing of urinary tract infections and their ability to reduce an enlarged prostate, though it is not understood how this works as yet.

Harvesting
Ripe berries are harvested in autumn, and the seeds are removed and then dried.

How to Use
An occasional infusion or a tincture of the dried berries can be taken as a general tonic, especially in the case of convalescence.

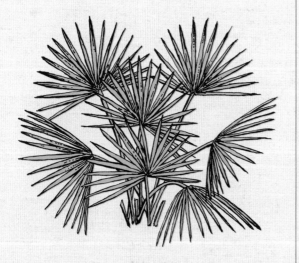

ORIGINS
Southwest Europe,
South Russia,
North Africa

SILYBUM MARIANUM (SYN. CARDUUS MARIANUS)

Milk thistle *Lady's thistle, marian thistle, blessed thistle*

Legend has it that the white markings on the leaves of the milk thistle plant are splashes of the Virgin Mary's milk. The seeds are a valuable source of winter food for birds such as goldfinches.

Caution
Milk thistle is a member of the Asteraceae family and should be avoided by anyone with a sensitivity to that plant group. Subject to control as a weed in some countries.

Cultivation
An annual or biennial that prefers well-drained soil in sun, milk thistle is hardy and will grow to around 1.2m (4ft) tall and 75cm (2½ft) wide.

A History of Healing
Gerard deemed milk thistle 'the best remedy that grows against all melancholy diseases' – melancholy at this time referred to an excess of black bile (that was not being cleared from the body by the liver), which caused physical as well as mental symptoms. Milk thistle's use in liver disorders dates back to at least Dioscorides in the 1st century CE, and its effectiveness has now been proven by modern trials. Compounds in the seeds have been shown to have a powerfully protective effect on the liver from damage from toxins as varied as the death cap mushroom, alcohol and chemotherapy drugs. Traditional Chinese medicine also uses milk thistle as a remedy for liver disorders such as cirrhosis. The seeds are known to be anti-inflammatory and an antioxidant.

Milk thistle was also considered a healthful spring vegetable, and was taken by breastfeeding mothers to increase milk production.

Harvesting
While the young flowerheads can be boiled and eaten in the same way as artichokes, it is the seeds that have the strongest therapeutic effect. Harvest these when they are ripe in late summer, removing the fluffy down, if necessary.

How to Use
Grind a teaspoonful of dried seeds, as needed, and sprinkle over food – they will not store once ground – during convalescence. Milk thistle can also help in the case of heavy alcohol consumption; eat a teaspoonful of seeds, ground over food or chewed directly, before going out and again the morning after, to protect the liver and help prevent a hangover.

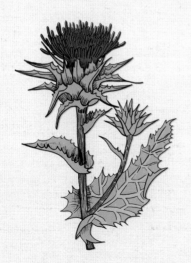

STELLARIA MEDIA

Chickweed *Star weed*

So named for its star-shaped flowers and popularity as a nutritious food for chickens and other fowl, chickweed is a common weed of the vegetable patch, but delicious in its own right.

Caution
Contraindicated during pregnancy.
Excessive consumption can have a laxative
and emetic effect.

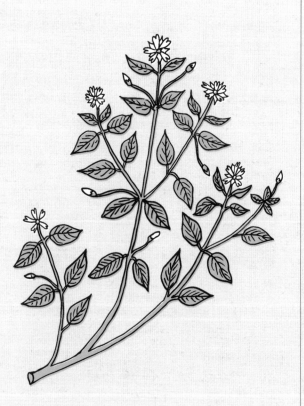

Cultivation
Chickweed has a long history of use for external complaints such as irritated eyes and itchy skin. Dioscorides recommended mixing chickweed with cornmeal and applying to the eyes; Hildegard of Bingen suggested that a warm poultice would help heal a person who had 'fallen by accident, or has been struck by cudgels, so that his skin is bruised'. Considered a cooling herb, chickweed is used to soothe inflamed and itchy skin, including nettle rash and sunburn. It is thought that an infusion can suppress the appetite when drunk before a meal, suggesting potential as a remedy for obesity.

Foraging
Pick the fresh parts as required. The juice can be frozen (mixed with aloe vera gel in an ice-cube tray, see page 78), but the plant does not dry well. Take care when foraging not to pick from any plant that might have been urinated on by dogs.

How to Use
Eat the leaves/stems/flowers fresh in salads. Drink a hot-water infusion to cleanse and soothe the digestion and dry/itchy skin. Once cooled, the infusion can be applied externally as an eyewash for dry, irritated eyes or as a compress for rashes and sunburn. The fresh aerial parts can also be applied as a poultice or added to a herbal bath; wilted aerial parts can be infused in oil and then used directly or mixed into balms.

SYMPHYTUM OFFICINALE

Comfrey *Knitbone, woundwort, bruisewort*

Culpeper wrote in the 17th century that comfrey was a 'very common but very neglected plant. It contains very great virtues,' a description that still applies today. It is also an excellent plant for bees and for making a nutritious 'tea' fertilizer for the garden.

Caution
Hairs on the leaves can be an irritant.
For external use only.

Cultivation
Comfrey is an invasive plant that is difficult to eradicate once grown. A hardy perennial, it prefers damp soil in full sun or partial shade, and will grow up to 1m (3ft) tall and 60cm (2ft) wide.

A History of Healing
Comfrey has been used for thousands of years as a wound-healer, both inside and out. It is so quick to promote skin healing that it is not recommended for deep cuts, as it can join the skin together on the surface before the deeper tissues have had a chance to heal, potentially

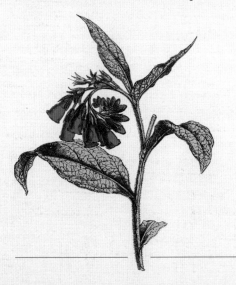

trapping infection and causing an abscess. Comfrey can also be used to promote the healing of muscular strains and sprains and broken bones. Culpeper even went so far as to repeat the legend that comfrey is so powerful a herb for knitting together wounds that if it was boiled in a pot with pieces of meat, it would cause them to join together again! The herb's healing properties come from its active constituent allantoin, which stimulates cells to proliferate and repair damaged tissue, and it also has anti-inflammatory properties. Its effects have been supported by evidence from trials showing faster recovery and healing for abrasions, sprains, bruises and back pain.

Historically, comfrey (both the leaf and the root) was also taken internally, but it is now known to contain high levels of toxic alkaloids that can cause liver damage if taken thus.

Harvesting
Pick the leaves in summer before the plant comes into flower, and use fresh or dry.

How to Use
The fresh leaves may be applied as a poultice or compress. Use fresh or dried leaves to make an infused oil or ointment to clean shallow wounds and grazes or place over inflamed joints or sprains. Make into a garden fertilizer (see page 36).

SYZYGIUM AROMATICUM
(SYN. *EUGENIA CARYOPHYLLATA*)

Clove

Cloves are the dried flower buds of this tree, picked twice a year and spread in the sun to dry. The flower buds contain the best essential oil, although the leaves and stems are sometimes used for oil distillation as well. From a very specific native of the Molucca Islands of Indonesia, cloves have spread across the world as a delicious culinary spice and useful medicinal herb.

Caution
Essential oil can cause dermatitis when applied to the skin.

Cultivation
The clove tree will reach 15–20m (49–66ft) in height and 3–5m (10–16½ft) in spread. It is evergreen, and needs a minimum temperature of 15–18°C (59–64°F), well-drained, rich soil and full sun.

A History of Healing
Cloves have been known for their value as a spice in the West for nearly two thousand years, where they are often associated with Christmas and studded orange pomanders. Aside from perhaps knowing a grandmother who sucked on a clove for toothache, they are widely undervalued as a therapeutic herb. Cloves reached China and India at around the same time, and became much more popular as a remedy in traditional Chinese medicine than they did in Ayurvedic healing, using cloves for a variety of complaints and viewing the plant as a panacea.

Clove oil contains a large proportion of eugenol, which is both strongly antiseptic and anaesthetic (making it an ideal choice for dentistry), and other compounds that are antispasmodic. Cloves are used to treat viral infections in tropical Asia; in India they are viewed as a warming, stimulating herb with aphrodisiac properties, and most Asian herbal medicines use cloves for digestive problems. Externally, cloves are used to heal skin complaints. Clove-studded oranges originated as insect repellents in the Moluccas.

How to Use
Use cloves whole or ground in cooking. Infuse whole cloves in hot water (perhaps mixed with other warming herbs such as ginger and cinnamon) to ease digestive discomfort, or prepare as a tincture. One or two drops of the essential oil can be rubbed onto a painful tooth. Whole cloves can be added to herbal sachets to use as moth repellents in linen cupboards.

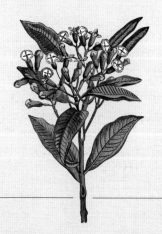

TABEBUIA IMPETIGINOSA (SYN. T. AVELLANEDAE)

Pau d'Arco *Lapacho, ipê-roxa*

Pau d'arco translates literally as 'bow-wood', referring to the durable timber's secondary use in making bows and arrows by the indigenous people of South America.

Caution
Seek professional medical advice before using pau d'arco if taking anticoagulant medication. Contraindicated during pregnancy and if trying to conceive. Excess can cause dizziness, vomiting and diarrhoea.

Cultivation
Pau d'arco needs a minimum temperature of 10–15°C (50–59°F), full sun and moist but well-drained soil. It is evergreen in its native habitat, but grown in colder climates it can be deciduous. It will reach up to 30m (98ft) tall and 15m (49ft) wide.

A History of Healing
Pau d'arco was the subject of much hope and expectation in the latter half of the last century as it underwent many clinical trials as a potential cancer treatment. It has known anticancer activity, and is also antibacterial and antifungal; it was used by the Incas and other South American peoples for complaints as varied as snake bites and dysentery for hundreds of years. However, although research has shown that the herb's constituents can suppress the growth of cancer cells, trials have yet to prove anything concretely positive.

Herbalists use pau d'arco as a natural antibiotic and antifungal (for example, against thrush) and a tonic herb for chronic fatigue syndrome, as well as to treat inflammatory conditions, especially of the digestive system.

Harvesting
It is the inner bark of the tree, stripped and dried, that is used for herbal preparations.

How to Use
Pau d'arco can be prepared as a decoction for an occasional tonic tea (it was reputedly favoured by Mahatma Ghandi) or to help clear thrush. A tincture can be taken over the longer-term to help with such conditions as chronic fatigue syndrome.

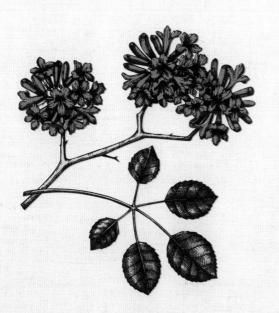

ORIGINS
Europe, Caucasia

TANACETUM PARTHENIUM

Feverfew *Featherfew, bachelor's buttons*

Feverfew is related to tansy (*T. vulgare*), a popular strewing herb with a strong insect-repelling essential oil and associations with Easter and Passover.

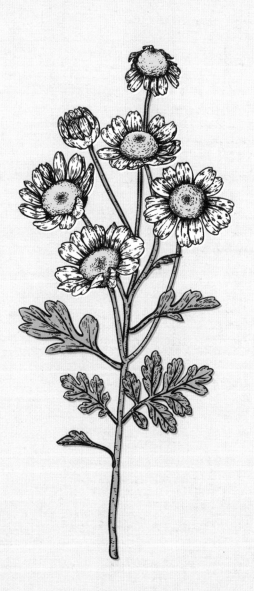

Caution
Contraindicated during pregnancy and for people taking aspirin and/or anticoagulant medication. Eating the fresh leaves and/or handling the plant can cause irritation to the mouth and skin in some people. A member of the Asteraceae family, it should be avoided by anyone with sensitivity to those plants.

Cultivation
Feverfew is a short-lived perennial that will easily seed around the garden if most of the flower heads are left on the plant; they can be used as cut flowers. Leave some to set seed to ensure future crops. It is herbaceous, reaching around 60cm (2ft) high and 30cm (12in) wide, and fully hardy. Grow in well-drained to dry soil in full sun.

A History of Healing

Although used as a therapeutic herb for hundreds of years, feverfew came to prominence as a migraine cure in the 1970s and 1980s. A lady called Anne Jenkins had suffered with migraines for 50 years, despite being married to a doctor, but after trying feverfew, she never experienced another. Scientific studies followed, and trials showed it was indeed effective when taken as a prophylactic remedy.

Prior to this, Parkinson had mentioned feverfew as a cure for headaches and fever, though as a poultice rather than being taken inwardly, but most medieval uses of the herb concentrated on childbirth and menstrual problems. It was also used as an antidote to excess opium consumption, and a remedy for dizziness, tinnitus and (because it is a bitter herb) taken as a digestive tonic. Feverfew has been researched for its potential in cases of rheumatoid arthritis, without definitive results, but it has been proven to have both anti-inflammatory and analgesic properties.

Harvesting

The leaves can be picked fresh as needed; the foliage will often persist on the plant in a mild winter. Culpeper wrote, 'And if any grumble because they cannot get the herb in winter, tell them, if they please, they may make a syrup of it in summer.'

How to Use

The fresh leaves can be eaten occasionally for the digestive benefit of their bitterness, or every day to help prevent migraines. Two or three leaves per day is considered enough for migraine prevention, and their bitterness will likely mean you won't want to add any more to a salad anyway. Add the leaves to a salad, chop and mix into butter with other herbs and spread onto bread (there is some suggestion the fats make the herb's active constituents more available to the body), or follow Parkinson's advice and fry them with eggs which, he says, are 'eaten with great delight; the bitternesse, which else would make it unpleasant, being taken away by the manner of dressing'. A tincture or syrup of the leaves can be prepared to use when fresh leaves are not available.

ORIGINS
Northern
hemisphere

TARAXACUM OFFICINALE

Dandelion *Lion's tooth, pissenlit, Pu Gong Ying*

Long known as a powerful diuretic, the French name *pissenlit* translates as 'wet-the-bed' or, according to Culpeper, 'piss-a-beds'. Fortunately it was the other French common name *dent-de-lion*, meaning 'lion's tooth', that was more prevalent and it is from that we now get the common name dandelion.

Caution
A member of the Asteraceae family, it should be avoided by people with sensitivity to these plants.

Cultivation
Dandelions can be a terrible weed – Elizabeth Blackwell wrote that 'it grows almost everywhere in Fallow Ground' – so remove the flower heads before they set seed. Grow in deep, sandy soil for easy harvesting of the roots but otherwise dandelions will grow in most soils in full sun. Hardy perennials, they will reach around 30cm (12in) in height and spread.

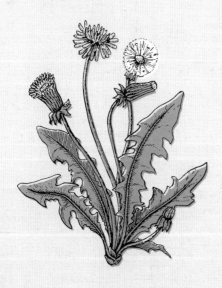

A History of Healing
These plants were and are viewed as a spring cleansing herb, taken to purify the blood and body of toxins and treat any associated (skin) conditions, as well as helping to clear excess fluid retention. Traditional Chinese medicine also uses dandelion as a cleansing herb to treat liver disorders and abscesses. The leaves are rich in potassium, so while other diuretics can cause a deficiency in it, dandelion rarely does.

Dandelion leaves are a valuable bitter herb and, according to Blackwell, are 'much eat as a Sallad in the Spring'. The roots are laxative, rich in prebiotic inulin and may have anticancer properties.

Foraging
Since they are ubiquitous and obvious, it is easy to find the leaves. There may well be local allotment and garden owners who would welcome an offer of having their dandelions dug up, which would mean that you can legally harvest the roots. The roots are best dug up in autumn, when they have a higher inulin content.

How to Use
Eat the young leaves raw or blanched in salads, or infuse fresh or dried leaves in hot water. Dried root can be decocted or roasted and ground as a coffee substitute.

THYMUS VULGARIS

Thyme *Garden thyme*

All garden thymes are excellent plants for bees; the honey they make from thyme flowers is delicious and beneficial. Thyme oil is also used to protect beehives against the devastating varroa mite. Wild thyme is not, as it would seem, a wild version of the garden thyme, but is in fact *T. serpyllum*, also known as creeping thyme and is an excellent plant for growing in the cracks of paving for a fragrant path; a tea of wild thyme was recorded by Mrs Grieve in her herbal as 'useful in the case of drunkeness'.

Caution
Essential oil is contraindicated for external use during pregnancy; avoid in large quantities while breastfeeding.

Cultivation
Grow in well-drained soil in full sun. Thymes are evergreen subshrubs that grow to around 25cm (10in) tall and 30cm (12in) wide. Cutting back the stems after flowering will keep plants from becoming straggly. Replace them every few years.

A History of Healing
A powerful yet gentle herb, 'it is so harmless you need not fear the use of it', wrote Culpeper. Thyme has antiseptic and antifungal qualities (due to a high proportion of eponymous thymol in its volatile oil) and has been used for almost every internal and external infection over the years, but especially in the case of bronchial infections. Parkinson recommended a decoction of thyme with honey, salt and vinegar when it could act as an expectorant 'to purge flegme'. It was also used for intestinal worms. Research has proven the antiseptic, antibacterial, antifungal and antioxidant properties of thyme and that it is effective in helping clear coughs and phlegm.

Harvesting
Regular picking will help keep the plant bushy and vibrant. Cut stems for drying as they begin to flower. Store dried stems whole and rub off the leaves as needed.

How to Use
Thyme is a delicious culinary herb with many applications, savoury and sweet. It can be infused in hot water for a tea to help relieve a cough or as a general digestive and immune system tonic. A cooled infusion mixed with honey makes a gargle for sore throats, or prepare as an oxymel. Thyme can be substituted for rosemary in a conditioning hair tonic that may encourage hair growth (see page 64).

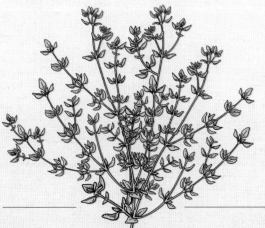

ORIGINS
East and Central
Europe

TILIA CORDATA (SYN. *T. PARVIFOLIA*)

Linden *Lime tree*

This lime tree bears no relation to the citrus fruit. It is often planted as a street tree, and is common enough in the countryside too, so foraging for the flowers in spring is easy. *Tilia* x *europaea*, *T. americana* and *T. platyphyllos* can be used interchangeably with *T. cordata*. The wood of the lime tree, which is much used for musical instruments, is especially valued for its lightness and ease of carving. The early 18th-century carvings attributed to Grinling Gibbons at Chatsworth House, Derbyshire, were made from lime wood.

Caution
Pollen can cause allergic reactions and hay fever in some people.

Cultivation
Limes form large deciduous trees up to 30–40m (98–131ft) tall, depending on the species, with a broad spread, and are fully hardy. *T. cordata* suckers less than other species but all are popular with aphids.

A History of Healing
Linden blossom has a lasting reputation as a relaxant and nerve tonic when drunk as an infusion or distilled water. An infusion will cause the drinker to perspire, and so it has also been used since medieval times as a gentle way to break a fever or to ward off the earliest signs of a cold. Mrs Grieve wrote in *A Modern Herbal* that 'prolonged baths prepared with the infused flowers are also good in hysteria.'

Foraging
Look for the flowers in spring – they bear a pale green bract, like a long, thin leaf or petal, to which the flowers are attached (this is to help the tree disperse its seeds once they are ripe; the bract acts as a sail in the wind). There is no need to separate the flowers from the bracts.

How to Use
Linden flowers make an uplifting and calming tisane, especially in the case of stress or anxiety; try them by themselves or mixed in equal quantities with St John's wort (see page 146) and lemon balm (see page 166). Drink plenty of fluids alongside to counteract the perspiration. Infuse the flowers in honey or a syrup. Scattered in a bedtime bath for adults or children, perhaps also with lavender (see page 156) and rose (see page 196), they will soothe and calm. The young leaves are edible.

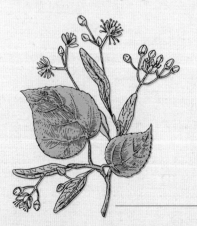

ORIGINS
Europe, except
extreme North
and South

TRIFOLIUM PRATENSE

Red clover *Trefoil*

The old saying to be 'in clover' means to be rich, referring to the clover plant's ability to fix nitrogen in the soil, thus enhancing the nutrient content of its meadow. It is therefore widely grown in pasture and as a green manure by gardeners.

It is thought that St Patrick used the three leaves (*tri-folium*) of the clover when teaching the people of Ireland about the Holy Trinity, though it is not known exactly which species was the inspiration for that or for the shamrock, Ireland's national symbol, or the origin of the inherent luck of a four-leaved clover.

Cultivation
Moist but well-drained soil in sun will suit clover best. It can be naturalized in a lawn, or grow the trailing variety 'Susan Smith' (syn. 'Dolly North') in a hanging basket or pot.

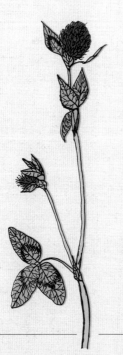

Clover is a hardy but short-lived perennial growing to 15cm (6in) high and around 45cm (18in) wide.

A History of Healing
Red clover is a traditional cleansing herb, helping to clear the lymph glands and skin in the case of eczema and psoriasis, and rich in minerals. Clover also contains phytoestrogens and is widely used to help balance the hormones and alleviate menopausal symptoms. It is also thought to protect the heart and bone density during the menopause.

In addition, clover has a reputation as a cure for cancer, which was touted during the 1930s. No clinical trials have been able to establish a benefit from red clover, but it is a gentle plant that herbalists recommend for its potential in both preventing and treating breast cancer.

Harvesting
Pick the flower heads as they start to open, taking the upper leaves as well, and dry before use. While it is possible to forage red clover from meadows, there is the risk of contamination from livestock, so it may be best to grow your own.

How to Use
Infuse the dried flower heads in hot water for a tisane to cleanse and/or help relieve hot flushes and breast pain.

TRIGONELLA FOENUM-GRAECUM

Fenugreek

The unusual triangular flowers and seeds of fenugreek inspired its genus
name, while the species name translates as 'Greek hay', referring to its use
as a supplementary fodder crop.

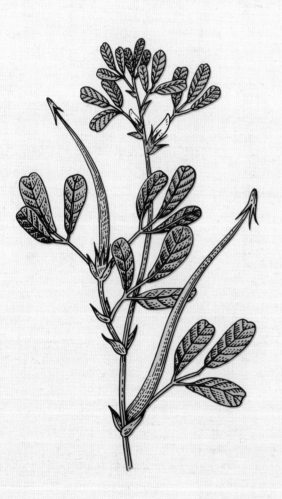

Caution
**Contraindicated during pregnancy and
hypoglycaemic therapy.**

Cultivation
Fenugreek is an annual with a height of 60cm
(2ft) and spread of around 35cm (14in).
It is frost tender, so crop indoors (see below)
or sow outside in late spring. It needs fertile,
well-drained soil in full sun.

A History of Healing
Fenugreek is a popular herb both for culinary
and therapeutic uses in the Middle East, Asia
and Mediterranean countries. It is known to
have been cultivated in Assyria nine thousand
years ago, there is evidence of its use in Iraq
from 4000 BCE, and it is mentioned in the
Ebers Papyrus from Ancient Egypt, *c.*1500 BCE.
In Western herbal traditions it was used
externally for burns and skin complaints and
internally (as recommended by Dioscorides)
for most gynaecological problems and to
induce childbirth.

The use of fenugreek in traditional Chinese medicine is as an overall tonic for the kidneys and to treat problems such as premature ejaculation and loss of libido, back pain and painful menstruation. Ayurveda uses fenugreek as an aphrodisiac and to treat a wide range of complaints, from digestive to bronchial, gout to arthritis.

Today, herbalists use fenugreek as an appetite stimulant during convalescence and in anorexia, as a soothing therapy for the digestion, and to encourage childbirth and breast-milk production. There is research interest in fenugreek's ability to lower blood cholesterol levels and stabilize blood sugar levels, which suggests that it may be of use in treating late-onset diabetes. The volume of seeds needed to achieve these effects is still unclear, but it is known that powdered seeds seem to have the best effect. Studies have shown that the seeds have antimicrobial and anti-inflammatory properties, and may have potential in treating liver cancer.

Tips for Growing

To sprout the seeds, put 1 teaspoon into a small glass jar and add some water. Leave overnight then drain off the water and put the jar on a sunny windowsill. Rinse the seeds in fresh water every day. The seeds will sprout a tiny root and shoot, and may be eaten at any stage from this point until when the first green growth appears. Alternatively, spread the seeds thickly in a shallow tray of potting compost or on a piece of damp kitchen towel. Keep them damp and once a dense crop of young leaves appears, snip them off to use as a garnish.

How to Use

Incorporate the seeds and seedlings into the diet, either lightly roasted then ground in foods and spice mixes, or as sprouted seeds or micro-veg. The fresh or dried leaves are also popular curry ingredients.

ORIGINS
South America

TROPAEOLUM MAJUS

Nasturtium

This salad herb is often used as a sacrificial companion plant in the vegetable patch, to attract blackfly away from bean crops, but its peppery leaves and flowers are tasty in their own right. The unripe seeds can be pickled in vinegar, and are known as 'poor man's capers'.

Cultivation
Sow seeds in spring and plant out after the last frost. Some cultivars of this tender annual trail or climb, while others have a bushier habit.

A History of Healing
Mainly used as a vitamin-rich salad herb, all parts of the nasturtium plant are now known to have antibiotic properties once ingested, increasing the body's resistance to infection. They can also have an expectorant effect, clearing phlegm and catarrh from the nose and airways.

Tips for Growing
Once infested with aphids, plants go quickly downhill, so nip off affected parts as soon as they are seen. Sow in succession through spring to ensure fresh plants take over once the first have gone to seed.

How to Use
Add the leaves and flowers to salads; pickle the seeds. A hot-water infusion of the leaves can help boost the immune system and clear a cold.

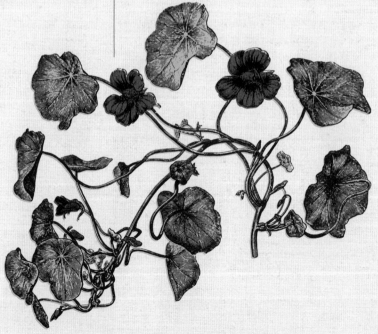

ORIGINS
East Asia

TURNERA DIFFUSA VAR. *APHRODISIACA* (SYN. *T. DIFFUSA*)

Damiana

A traditional tonic herb and aphrodisiac used by the Mayan culture in Central America, damiana extract is also used to make Damiana, a Cointreau-like liqueur.

Cultivation

Damiana is a half-hardy shrub that grows 1–2m (3–6½ft) in height and 60cm (2ft) in spread. Grow in dry soil in full sun and cut back in spring.

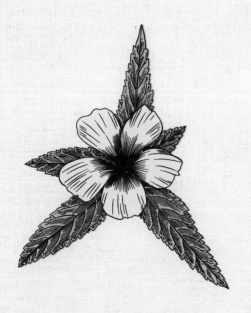

A History of Healing

As a tonic, damiana is used as a restorative for cases of nervous exhaustion and mild depression and anxiety. Reputed to affect testosterone levels, stimulating the libido for both men and women, it is regarded as a helpful herb for impotence and delayed periods. Damiana is known to contain the antiseptic and tonic constituent thymol and also arbutin, a substance that is converted in the body into a urinary antiseptic. Finally, damiana is used as a mild laxative.

Clinical trials have yet to prove definitively the aphrodisiac effects of damiana, though there have been positive results in tests on rats. Research has had encouraging results vis-à-vis its antidepressant action and antibacterial effect on bladder infections, and studies also show that the herb may lower blood sugar levels and be of use in treating diabetes.

Harvesting

The leaves of the plant are harvested in summer, when the plant is flowering, and dried to use in infusions and proprietary preparations such as tablets.

How to Use

A tincture of the leaves can be taken as a tonic and antidepressant; a small cup of tisane can also be taken as a general tonic and to relieve urinary infections.

ULMUS RUBRA (SYN. *U. FULVA*)

Slippery elm *Red elm, moose elm*

Although the most effective elm for therapeutic use is the slippery elm, the white elm (*U. americana*) was used in a similar way in North America. Across the Atlantic, the inner bark of native European elms was also used as a demulcent herb. The outer bark of the slippery elm has an unsavoury history as an abortifacient of mixed-race foetuses from North America and is now banned in many countries. The inner bark has no such effect.

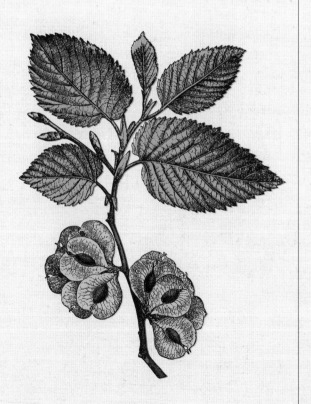

Cultivation

Deep, moist soil in full sun will best suit slippery elm, which can grow to a height and spread of around 20m (66ft). It is a fully hardy deciduous tree, but may succumb to Dutch elm disease.

A History of Healing

The inner bark of slippery elm is made up of a large proportion of mucilage, which has a soothing effect on inflamed membranes in many parts of the body. The use of elms as a demulcent was first mentioned by Dioscorides in the 1st century CE, and although there has been little clinical research, the effects of the demulcent are well understood.

Slippery elm powder can be mixed with water, with added honey and spices such as nutmeg and cinnamon (see page 108), to form a thin, prebiotic gruel which is an excellent gentle and nutritious food for babies and convalescents. When the herb is used for inflammation, it coats the irritated membranes, soothing them and drawing out any toxins. It can thus be used to relieve bronchial and chest infections, acid reflux and gastrointestinal problems, alleviating diverticulitis, gastroenteritis and other inflammations of the gut and helping both constipation and diarrhoea (making it useful for irritable bowel syndrome). Applied externally as a poultice to inflamed areas, slippery elm can draw out boils, splinters and other skin infections, while calming and softening the skin.

Harvesting

The inner bark is the only part of the slippery elm that is used. Mrs Grieve reported in her herbal that large quantities of the bark are collected from ten-year-old trees, and 'as the wood has no commercial value, the tree is fully stripped and consequently dies'. Trees are now rare in the wild. The bark is dried and often powdered before use.

How to Use

Slippery elm powder can be mixed with warm water to help alleviate gastrointestinal problems, coughs and acid reflux. Alternatively, mix the powder with honey (in roughly equal quantities, but adjust to get the right consistency) and roll into pastilles that can be stored in an airtight jar for up to six months, to be eaten whenever the symptoms of acid reflux or acid in the stomach strike. Mixed into a paste with a small quantity of aloe vera gel (see page 78), adding a few drops of lavender essential oil, if liked (see page 156), the powder can be applied as a poultice for stings and boils.

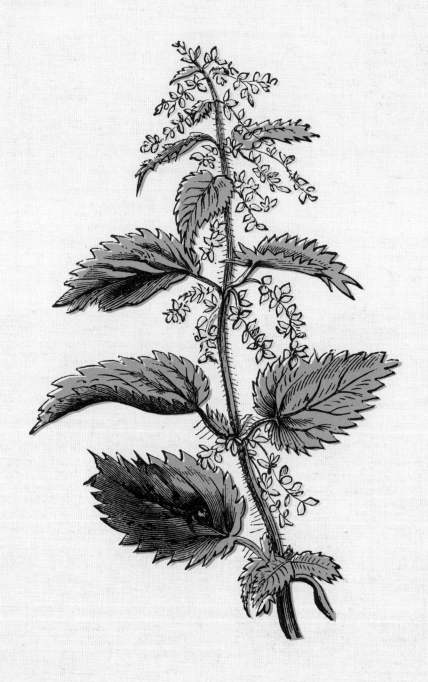

URTICA DIOICA

Nettle *Stinging nettle*

Nettles are usually considered the bane of both gardens and country walks: they are persistent, difficult to eradicate and deliver a painful sting. However, they are in fact an incredibly useful plant – they provide nutritious food and therapeutic qualities, and can also be used as a dye and cloth plant. Nettles are also particularly useful for wildlife and attract beneficial insects such as ladybirds to the garden where they prey on garden pests. Combine the nettle's assets with the fact they need next to no encouragement to grow, and it is perhaps time to see them in a new light.

Caution
Excess can cause a build-up of toxins in the body and a rash.

Cultivation
Most would prefer not to cultivate nettles in their garden, for, as Elizabeth Blackwell pointed out, 'The Nettle grows everywhere in too great Plenty.' However, they are a valuable herb and crop, and also a wonderful plant for wildlife (especially butterflies, such as the red admiral), so it is worth letting a small patch, or stand, grow if possible. They prefer moist, rich soil in sun or dappled shade. Pull up the smaller plants around the edge of the stand to prevent them spreading by running roots, and cut some down in late spring for a fresh flush of leaves, leaving the rest for the wildlife.

A History of Healing
Britain has the Romans to thank for the introduction of the nettle to these shores; they would deliberately sting themselves all over to stimulate the circulation and help them warm up in cold winters ('urtication'). Although it would seem like needless suffering, deliberate stinging is still employed by some as a topical rubefacient to alleviate even more painful conditions such as arthritis, though there is little clinical evidence to support this. Nettles can be used as an anti-allergenic; the topical application of the juice is the best remedy for the stings caused by its own leaves, and an infusion is a traditional hay-fever cure.

There is some evidence from trials that taking the roots may help with the urinary difficulties caused by an enlarged prostate (BPH). Nettles are a diuretic, and one of the spring cleansing herbs when drunk as an infusion, and useful for skin conditions and arthritis. Nettles are also beneficial for the hair, treating dandruff and adding body and shine. A medieval cosmetic custom was to dip one's comb in nettle juice before backcombing the hair to encourage its growth. Dioscorides also recommended nettle as an astringent, good for stopping a nosebleed.

The nettle 'is one of the few wild herbs still gathered each spring by country-folk as a pot-herb. It makes a healthy vegetable, easy of digestion,' wrote Mrs Grieve in her herbal. The leaves are rich in vitamins, minerals and fibre, although overconsumption of the leaves (including as an infusion) can lead to a rash. The seeds are an antioxidant and were held by Parkinson to be an excellent countermeasure for lethargy.

The name nettle derives from the Anglo-Saxon *noedl*, needle. This may refer to the stings, (as with *Urtica* - from the Latin *urere* 'to burn') but is probably referring to the fact that the fibres of the plant were used to weave fabric and fishing nets. Other textile plants, such as hemp and flax, eventually took the place of nettles but they came back into use during both world wars, for example, to make German army uniforms.

Foraging

Culpeper had this advice for nettle foragers, which can also help distinguish nettles from the dead nettle (*Lamium album*): 'they may be found by feeling'. Wear rubber or other thick gloves and suitable clothing to avoid the stings, said to be the tines of the Devil's pitchfork in Irish mythology. Gather nettles in early to mid-spring, when their growth is fresh and green, and pick off the top four to six sets of leaves. Do not pick once the plant is flowering, although where nettles are cut back, there may be a second crop of young leaves to be had later in the year. Cut some to dry as well; they can still sting after drying. Older plants can be hung upside down in a paper bag to catch the seeds. Eat the seeds fresh or freeze to preserve them, as they do not dry well.

How to Use

Infuse fresh or dried leaves in hot water for a cleansing tea; combine with elderflower or chamomile to help prevent hay fever. An infusion can also be used as a final rinse for the hair after washing. Dried, crumbled leaves can be sprinkled (use a spoon!) into sauces as they cook to add some extra vitamins. Eat the seeds directly, or sprinkle over cereal or porridge.

NETTLE SOUP *serves 2*

Use the fresh leaves as you would spinach, blanching them (raw leaves, even crushed, can be an internal irritant) only briefly to remove the stings and preserve as much of the nutritional benefit as possible.

1 onion

2 garlic cloves

olive oil or butter

1 potato, peeled and roughly chopped

1 carrot, peeled and roughly chopped

1 litre (1¾ pints) vegetable stock

bunch of nettles, leaves picked and blanched (see above)

2 tablespoons crème fraiche or single cream

salt and black pepper

Fry the onion and garlic in butter or oil in a large saucepan over a gentle heat for a few minutes until softened, but not browned.

Add the chopped potato and carrot and cook for a few minutes before adding the vegetable stock. Simmer until the vegetables are tender, then add the blanched nettles and stir for a couple of minutes.

Transfer the soup to a blender, or use an electric hand blender, and process until smooth. Stir in the crème fraiche or cream, if liked, and season with salt and pepper to taste before serving.

ORIGINS
Europe to
North Asia

VACCINIUM MYRTILLUS

Bilberry *Winberry, huckleberry, whortleberry*

Bilberries are the wild ancestor of blueberries, and related to cranberries (*Vaccinium macrocarpon*), which have a powerful antibacterial action on the urinary tract, helping especially in cases of cystitis.

Caution
Take medical advice before using bilberries in significant doses (for example, tablets) if also using anticoagulant medication.

Cultivation
Bilberries are hardy, low-growing, deciduous shrubs, reaching 45cm (18in) in height and spreading indefinitely. They are often found on heathland and hillsides, but dislike alkaline (lime) soils, and will grow in sun or partial shade.

A History of Healing
Bilberries have a high concentration of anthocyanins in their fruit, more so than blueberries which have been bred over the years to produce larger, sweeter fruit at the expense of the intense blue-purple colouring that is so nutritious. Anthocyanins are beneficial for the circulation; trials have proven the effectiveness of bilberries in protecting and improving the

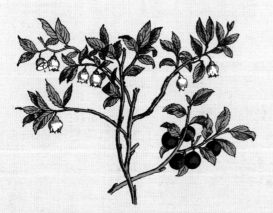

circulation, especially to the extremities and micro-capillaries. This, in turn, helps with symptoms of poor blood flow, such as regular pins and needles, cramps and fluid retention. During the Second World War, pilots noticed that the bilberry jam they were eating helped them see in the dark. Subsequent research has shown that the improved circulatory effect of the berries helps strengthen the eyes as well, stimulating the retina to see more clearly, especially in dim light.

The antioxidant properties of bilberries help repair and protect the body's tissues, which means they can help protect against heart disease, degenerative diseases and cancer. One trial of bilberry extract showed it to protect normal colon cells but to inhibit the growth of colon cancer cells, making them of significant interest in cancer treatment research. Like cranberries, bilberries can also help alleviate cystitis and other urinary tract infections. The leaves may have potential in treating the early stages of diabetes.

Harvesting
Fruits will be ripe in late summer to early autumn; leaves can be picked in summer.

How to Use
Add the fruits – fresh or dried – to food. Fresh fruits can be frozen or preserved as jam to eat out of season.

VALERIANA OFFICINALIS

Valerian *Common valerian, garden valerian, garden heliotrope*

Valerian also lends its common name to red valerian, *Centranthus ruber*, which is no relation and has no therapeutic value.

Caution
Contraindicated in conjunction with other sleep-inducing drugs and antidepressants. Can cause drowsiness.

Cultivation
Valerian prefers moist soil, but will grow in sun or partial shade. It is a hardy perennial and reaches a height and spread of around 1–1.5m (3–5ft). To encourage bigger rhizomes, cut off the flowers as they appear.

A History of Healing
Valerian's history as a sedative dates back to Hippocrates; Galen recommends it as a cure for insomnia. Anglo-Saxon and medieval herbals all mention valerian, and it was in the Middle Ages when it acquired the name all-heal. It was known as an effective remedy for epilepsy, and remained the primary treatment for that condition until the 19th century. Valerian was also used to alleviate the symptoms of other nervous conditions and it is now known that its effectiveness is due to how it affects the way chemical messages are sent in the brain: it regulates and slows the nervous system, especially helping those prone to overthinking and worrying.

It is of particular use to people suffering from anxiety and what Mrs Grieve in her herbal calls 'nervous overstrain', and it was given to soldiers with shellshock during the First World War. Valerian's great advantage over other drugs is that it has no discernible side-effects and is not addictive; it is calming, rather than sedative, and by lowering the stress level, it can also lower stress-related high blood pressure. As a muscle-relaxant it can help with tension in the neck and shoulders, period pain and irritable bowel syndrome.

Harvesting
Lift the rhizomes in the autumn (after the leaves have died back) to use fresh or dry. Leave new plants to establish for two years before harvesting.

How to Use
Prepare the root as a tincture to help alleviate anxiety. To calm, relax and aid sleep, take as a decoction (up to 100ml/7 tbsp) at night, or incorporate in a relaxing tisane mix (see page 44).

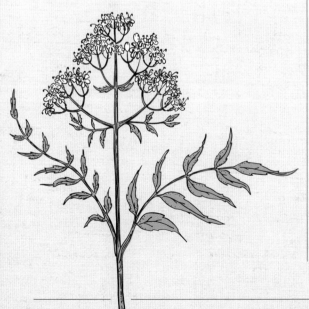

VERBENA OFFICINALIS

Vervain *Verbena, Ma Bian Cao*

ORIGINS
Europe,
West Asia,
North Africa

Vervain was once revered as a magical plant, held in high esteem by the Druids, Romans and other ancient civilizations. It was used in love potions and carried as a talisman against witchcraft and sorcery (Gerard called this 'vaine and superstitious'). The flowers are less showy than some of the ornamental species, such as *V. bonariensis*, but vervain still makes a fine plant for the border. *V. hastata* can be used interchangeably with *V. officinalis*.

Caution
Contraindicated during pregnancy.
Excess causes vomiting.

Cultivation
Vervain needs a sunny position and moist but well-drained soil. It is a hardy perennial that grows to 75cm (2½ft) tall and 60cm (2ft) wide.

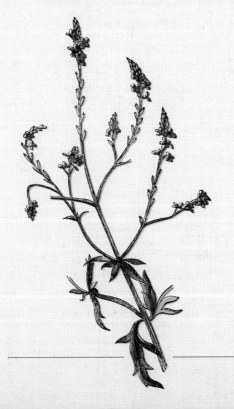

A History of Healing
Called a 'sacred herb' by Dioscorides, vervain was taken as a cure-all for many centuries. It is viewed as a tonic for the digestion and nervous systems, as a cure for coughs and colds, and a remedy for all nervous and stress-related symptoms, such as headaches and anxiety. Herbalists in both Western traditions and traditional Chinese medicine use vervain for anxiety, mild depression and long-term stress and the symptoms they cause. As a bitter herb, it can be beneficial for the digestion.

Research has so far shown some antiviral and sedative effects, and that vervain may be anti-inflammatory and protect nerve cells. Verbenalin, one of the plant's active constituents, is strongly bitter and can cause contractions of the womb and vomiting in excess.

Harvesting
Cut the plant down as flowering begins, and use fresh or dry, to store.

How to Use
Add to hot-water infusions to steady the nerves and ease premenstrual tension, anxiety, low mood, headaches and digestive cramps.

VIBURNUM OPULUS

Cramp bark *Guelder rose*

A common hedgerow shrub, cramp bark has scarlet, translucent, extremely smelly berries that are unpalatable for human consumption but loved by birds. The bark of the related *Viburnum prunifolium* (black haw, American sloe) is thought to have an antispasmodic activity and was traditionally used to prevent miscarriage and relieve morning sickness in pregnancy.

Caution
Contraindicated in the case of sensitivity to aspirin and salicylates.

Cultivation
Cramp bark is a deciduous shrub that will grow in partial shade or full sun and prefers a deep, moist soil. It will reach 5m (16½ft) tall and 4m (13ft) wide unless regularly pruned as part of a hedge.

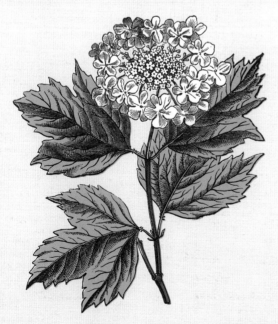

A History of Healing
There has been little research into cramp bark, but it and its North American cousin black haw both have a long history of use as remedies for cramps and muscle pains all over the body. This suggests it is of use for back and shoulder pain, night cramps, period pain, asthma and arthritis, or any other condition causing over-contraction of the muscles.

Harvesting
Cut the stems just before leaf fall in autumn or just before bud burst in spring, and strip off the bark to dry.

How to Use
Prepare the dried bark as a tincture or a decoction. For period pain and long-term conditions, herbalists recommend taking a tincture of cramp bark regularly throughout the month for the best results. Taking a tincture only when suffering the pain will have little to no effect, but a decoction may help. The dried bark can also be infused into an oil that is massaged into the affected areas.

VITEX AGNUS-CASTUS

Chaste-tree *Monk's pepper*

In Ancient Greece, the blue and white flowers and the branches of the chaste tree were woven into headdresses and worn by the virginal priestesses of Ceres. Priests and other celibates down the ages have taken the herb to cool sexual desire.

Caution
Contraindicated during pregnancy and when taking contraceptive medication or fertility treatments. Excess can cause an itchy skin (formication), and in rare cases an allergic reaction may occur, causing stomach upset, dizziness and/or headaches.

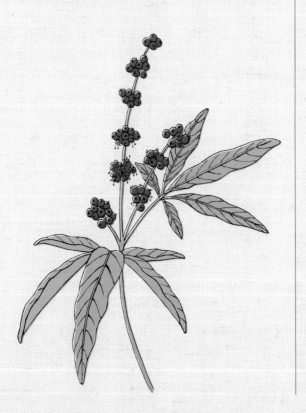

Cultivation
The chaste tree is actually a shrub growing to a height and spread of up to 2–8m (6½–26ft). It is frost hardy and deciduous, and prefers a well-drained or even poor soil. Prune the previous year's growth back to two buds in spring.

A History of Healing
The chaste tree was mentioned in Homer's Iliad (6th century BCE) as a plant capable of warding off evil, including temptations of the flesh. The seeds, ground and used as a condiment, were taken by monks as an anaphrodisiac, hence the common name monk's pepper.

   Today, the herb is known to have an effect on the hormones and neurotransmitters in the brain, leading to improved sleep (especially where melatonin levels are affected by jet lag and night-shift working) and a better-regulated menstrual cycle, also reducing related symptoms such as irritability, acne and breast tenderness. It is also thought to increase fertility where low progesterone levels are a problem. In men it can be a remedy for premature ejaculation.

Harvesting
The berries are harvested in autumn and dried.

How to Use
The dried, ground berries can be used in spice mixes. Proprietary tablets are available for premenstrual syndrome relief.

WITHANIA SOMNIFERA

Ashwagandha *Indian ginseng, winter cherry*

Ashwagandha is the Ayurvedic equivalent of ginseng (see page 178) in traditional Chinese medicine, an adaptogenic herb and overall tonic for a healthy, long life. It is also used in Middle Eastern and African herbal traditions to treat a wide range of conditions.

Caution
Toxic to animals.

Cultivation
A frost-hardy, evergreen shrub of variable size – 60cm–2m (2–6½ft) in height, 30cm–1m (1–3ft) in spread – that grows on dry, stony soil in full sun or partial shade.

A History of Healing
Most of ashwagandha's tonic and adaptogenic traditional uses have been supported by clinical studies. It is known to contain compounds

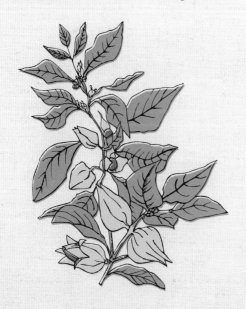

similar to the steroid hormones produced by the body, and seems to lower overall stress levels, bringing down levels of the stress hormone cortisol as well as stress-related high blood pressure. Ashwagandha can reduce anxiety and fatigue and increase concentration, memory and general well-being; it is used as a rejuvenating tonic in old age and during convalescence. It is also used for a better quality of sleep, as the *somnifera* part of its name suggests. Ashwagandha is high in iron and can therefore assist in recovery from anaemia.

Harvesting
Roots and fruits are harvested in autumn, the leaves in spring. Dry the roots before use.

How to Use
A decoction of the dried root can be drunk in small quantities to relieve stress and its associated symptoms – herbalists suggest 5g (2 tbsp) decocted in 100ml (7 tbsp) of water taken over two days. Ayurvedic remedies usually decoct ashwagandha root in milk, often with honey or sugar and/or rice. It is also available to buy as a powder, either loose or in capsule form. Sprinkle the loose powder over food in small quantities of ½–1 teaspoon per serving; try adding it to Bircher muesli or porridge just before serving, for example.

ORIGINS
Tropical Asia

ZINGIBER OFFICINALE

Ginger

Anyone who has ever eaten a ginger biscuit or had a cup of ginger tea to assuage nausea knows the incredible benefit this herb has on the digestion. Ginger is widely used as a culinary spice and a therapeutic herb. Around half of all preparations in both Ayurvedic and traditional Chinese medicine involve ginger; in Ayurvedic medicine, ginger is known as *vishwabhesaj*, the universal medicine.

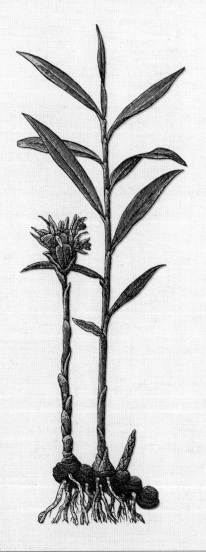

Caution
Contraindicated in therapeutic doses in the case of peptic ulcers and when taking anticoagulant medicines. During pregnancy, herbalists recommend no more than 2g (½ teaspoon) dried or 4g (1 teaspoon) fresh root per day.

Cultivation
Ginger needs high humidity and a minimum temperature of 10°C (50°F). It grows best in well-drained, rich soil in sun or partial shade, but can be grown in a large, wide pot as a house plant or in a greenhouse.

A History of Healing
Dioscorides described ginger as being 'right good with meat in sauces'. Ginger is widely used as a remedy for all forms of nausea and sickness, such as morning and motion sickness, and this use is backed up by extensive clinical evidence. It also has antiseptic and antimicrobial properties, so can assist in gastrointestinal infections and food poisoning. Ginger is seen as an overall digestive tonic to strengthen a weakened digestion, especially in the elderly and convalescents.

Ginger is a warming and stimulating herb, comforting and boosting the circulation, helping to clear cold and colds, and warming the hands and feet either when drunk as an infusion or eaten, or when massaged into the skin as an infused oil. As an anti-inflammatory, ginger has been shown to reduce muscle pain after exercise and, when taken regularly, can relieve period pains.

Harvesting

Although ginger can make a good house plant, heavy harvests of the rhizome may not be possible, so buy the rhizomes and use the plant for the leaves instead. Wrap the larger leaves around fish, meat or vegetables when baking or barbequing, to impart a gentle spice to the contents. The smaller leaves and young shoots are slightly spicy and can be added to curries and other dishes, or wilted and pureed to make a green sauce.

The oldest rhizomes can be removed after around ten months of growth, once new shoots have appeared.

How to Use

Infuse the fresh rhizome in hot water for a warming drink that will also calm the digestion and nausea or help to head off a cold – add lemon, honey and/or other herbs, if liked. All forms of ginger can be used in cooking and baking; crystallized ginger can be nibbled on directly as a snack.

FORMS OF GINGER

Dried ground ginger, as used in spice mixes for culinary use, is made from the dried and powdered rhizome. On drying, the chemical compounds in ginger that give it its characteristic taste and smell (known as gingerols) break down into different compounds called shoagols that are twice as hot and spicy as the gingerols.

Fresh ginger is the lifted rhizomes, although the rhizomes are actually no longer truly fresh by the time they reach the shops. By then, they will have dried out significantly and developed a thick skin, and taste quite different from the just-harvested young rhizome. This needs no peeling, and is sometimes called 'green ginger', although, confusingly, the name is also used to describe fresh ginger.

Crystallized ginger is made by boiling the fresh rhizome in a sugar syrup (see page 248). Stem ginger in syrup is also the fresh rhizome cooked in syrup, but instead of removing the ginger, it is stored in the cooking syrup, which keeps it softer. Gari is a pickled ginger used in Japanese cuisine.

STEM GINGER IN SYRUP AND CRYSTALLIZED GINGER

Both of these preserves are easy to make, for a ready store of ginger or a lovely home-made gift. Makes around one small jam jar of either type.

200g fresh ginger rhizome

200g (1 cup) golden caster sugar

65g (3 tbsp) honey

For stem ginger in syrup: Freeze the ginger for 24 hours to soften the fibres. Remove from the freezer, peel and cut into medium-sized chunks. Put into a saucepan and just cover with water, then simmer for around 1 hour until the ginger is soft to the point of a knife. Add around one-third of the sugar, stir until dissolved and then simmer for 10 minutes. Remove from the heat and leave to stand for 2–3 hours. Add half the remaining sugar, put the pan back on the heat and stir to dissolve, then simmer for 10 minutes. Remove from the heat and again leave to stand for 2–3 hours. Repeat with the final batch of sugar, this time simmering until the liquid is a thick syrup, add the honey and bring to the boil before transferring into a warm sterilized jar and seal.

For crystallized ginger: Follow the steps above, but cut the ginger into smaller pieces. After adding the honey and bringing it to the boil, pour the contents of the pan over a wire rack set over a tray to catch the dripping syrup. Leave to drain and dry, then roll in golden caster sugar before storing in an airtight jar. The syrup is no longer needed, but delicious in its own right and can be added to a tisane of mint, or drizzled over a cake, porridge or pancakes.

GLOSSARY

ACTIVE CONSTITUENT The part of the herb that has a healing effect

ADAPTOGEN A herb or active constituent of a herb that has the general effect on the body of boosting immunity and the ability to adapt to change, and increase resistance to external stressors

ALKALOID A member of a large group of chemicals found naturally in plants, often having diverse and important physiological effects on humans

ANALGESIC A herb or medicine that eases pain

ANNUAL A plant that lives and dies within a year

ANTI-INFLAMMATORY Something that reduces inflammation (swelling)

ANTIFUNGAL Something that inhibits fungal growth

ANTIHISTAMINE A substance that eases allergic reactions and/or reduces their symptoms

ANTIOXIDANT A substance that lessens the damaging effect of oxidization and free radical damage to the body

AROMATIC Rich in fragrant oils

ASTRINGENT Something that causes body tissues to contract, often due to a high tannin content

BIENNIAL A plant that flowers and sets seed in its second year

BITTER A bitter-tasting herb that aids digestion; **BITTERS** A remedy made from these herbs, typically a tincture. Also used as cocktail flavourings

CALYX (CALYCES) Part of the flower surrounding the petals

CARMINATIVE Something that eases intestinal bloating and gas and reduces griping

CARRIER OIL Oil used to dilute an essential oil

CONTRAINDICATION/ CONTRAINDICATED When a herb is not recommended for a specific condition or life stage, such as during pregnancy

DAMPING OFF Collapse of seedlings in conditions of extreme moisture

DECOCTION Hot-water infusion using tough plant materials, such as bark

DECONGESTANT A substance that helps to ease nasal and upper respiratory tract congestion/mucus and catarrh

DEMULCENT The mucilaginous property of a herb that is soothing to irritation or inflammation

DIAPHORETIC A substance that promotes perspiration

DIURETIC Something that increases the production of urine and/or its elimination

DOCTRINE OF SIGNATURES Herbal system based on the idea that God marked plants to resemble the parts of the body that they should be used to heal

ESSENTIAL OIL An oil made by distilling herbs, unsuitable for culinary use or other consumption

EXPECTORANT Something that aids the bringing up of catarrh when coughing

FLAVONOID An organic compound that occurs as a pigment in fruit and flowers

GENUS A class of similar plants

HYPOTENSIVE A substance that aids the lowering of blood pressure

INULIN Prebiotic that promotes healthy gut flora

OXYMEL Syrup containing a mix of herbs, sugar and vinegar

PERENNIAL Plant that can continue to grow for at least two years

PHYTOESTROGEN Plant-derived dietary oestrogen

PHYTOPHOTOTOXICITY When a plant (usually the sap) reacts with the skin and sunlight to produce a rash or irritation

PHYTOTOXIC Toxic to plants

PREBIOTIC A food that promotes the growth of beneficial digestive bacteria

QI Life force in traditional Chinese medicine

RHIZOME Horizontal stem from which a plant may grow

RUBEFACIENT An application that increases blood flow to the skin, also causing it to redden

SALICYLIC ACID A substance used in the manufacture of aspirin

SEDATIVE A substance that calms and induces sleep

SPECIES Group of plants within a genus

STYPTIC Something that helps to stop the flow of blood from a wound

SYN. Abbreviation of 'synonym', indicating an alternative name for a plant

TONIC A restorative remedy that tones and strengthens either a specific bodily system, such as the digestion, or the whole body

TCM Traditional Chinese medicine

VOLATILE OIL Another name for **ESSENTIAL OIL**, volatile oils typically are released from a plant's leaves through touch or evaporation, creating a fragrance

INDEX

PICTURE CREDITS

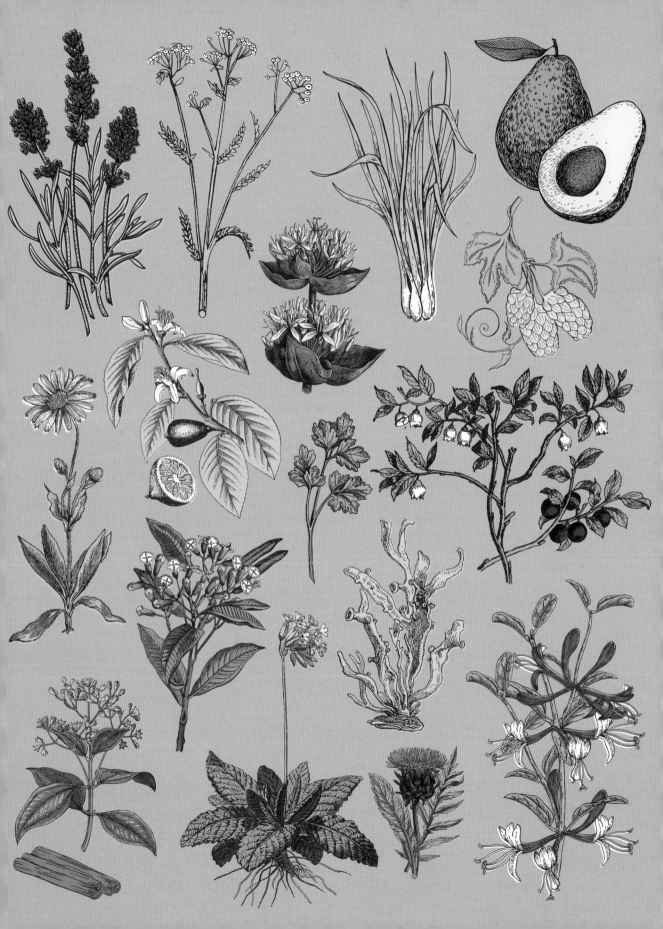

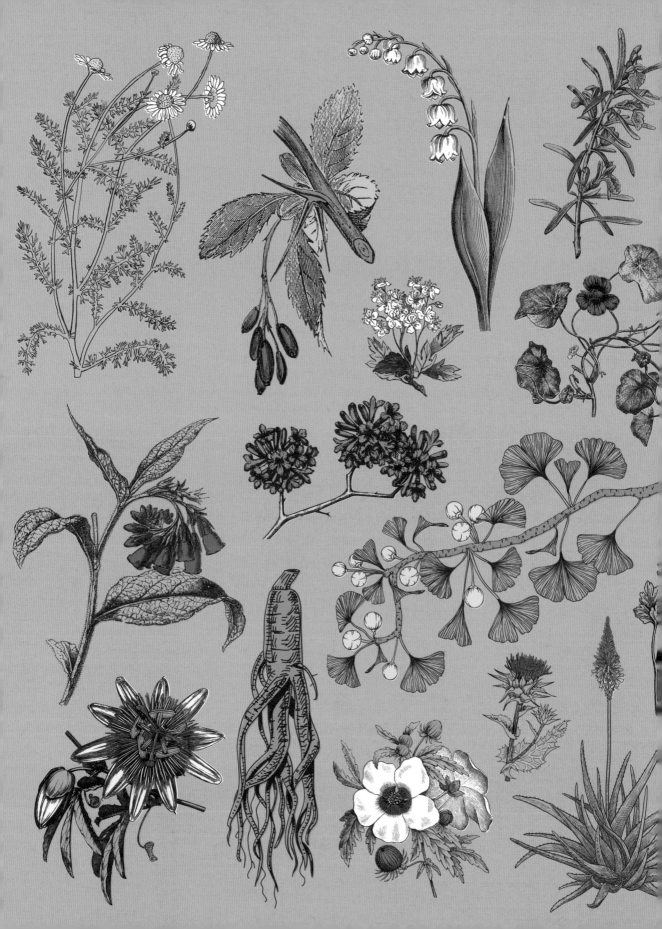